T0195428

ICU

QUICK D_____G GUI__

ICU

QUICK DRUG GUIDE

Editor

Jennifer Pai Lee, Pharm.D., BCPS

http://icuquickdrug.com

Elsevier
1600 John F. Kennedy Blvd.
Ste 1800
Philadelphia, PA 19103-2899

ICU QUICK DRUG GUIDE, FIRST EDITION   ISBN: 978-0-323-68047-9

Library of Congress Control Number: 2020936545

Content Strategist: Sara Watkins
Content Development Specialist: Michael Houston
Publishing Services Manager: Deepthi Unni
Project Manager: Radjan Lourde Selvanadin
Design Direction: Amy Buxton

Printed in India

Last digit is the print number: 9   8   7   6   5   4   3

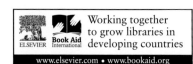

To my soul mate, Joseph, and endearing angels,
Jonathan and Joshua.

Foreword

The use of multiple pharmacologic interventions in patients in critical care scenarios requires an in-depth background and often a quick reference source. Working in the intensive care unit (ICU) as a pharmacist for many years, Dr. Lee identified the need for the quick reference to make our significant pharmacologic interventions as accurate and easy as possible. With this goal in mind and as part of her need to help the patients and their care providers, she created the *ICU Quick Drug Guide* reference book.

The *ICU Quick Drug Guide* is remarkable in its scope and detail. It is clearly organized and arranged to cover nearly all possible scenarios of the critically ill patients who may cross the doors of the ICU. The book is divided into six sections covering 24 different specific critical scenarios. Each chapter is divided into a brief discussion of drugs used for the specific treatment of the condition and clinical scenario. It is presented in an outline format accompanied by numerous clear descriptive tables of drug dosing, alternative agents, their antidotes (if available), potential complications, and drug interactions that may be encountered.

For the ICU nurses, residents, and physicians alike, this book will become an invaluable reference. For ICU teams rounding together, it will answer questions rapidly and accurately. I can find no other similar reference in medicine and believe that the *ICU Quick Drug Guide* will become a standard in the industry.

On a personal note, it was my pleasure to assist Dr. Lee in her pursuit of her career goals beyond her initial research studies on drugs for critically ill patients, particularly those involving renal failure and spinal cord injury. Jennifer has devoted her time and training toward the betterment of patients through education and understanding of how our drugs work, in whom they best work, and in what circumstances problems with our drugs may be anticipated or avoided. I believe all readers will find this book useful and a highly valuable resource.

Morton J. Kern, MD, MSCAI, FAHA, FACC
Chief of Medicine, VA Long Beach Health Care System
Professor of Medicine, University of California, Irvine

About the Author

Jennifer Pai Lee received her Doctorate of Pharmacy from the University of Southern California School of Pharmacy in 2001. Following graduation, she completed a residency in Clinical Pharmacy Practice at the Long Beach Memorial Medical Center in 2002. She is a Board Certified Pharmacotherapy Specialist and serves as an clinical faculty at University of California San Francisco, University of the Pacific, and University of Southern California Schools of Pharmacy. She has been teaching medical and pharmacy students and residents for almost twenty years as a clinical pharmacist in critical care. Her practice interests include pharmacokinetics, critical care medicine, and cardiology.

Jennifer is currently the Program Manager for Critical Care/Emergency Services at Veterans Affairs Long Beach Healthcare System. She has developed numerous guidelines and protocols that are essential in taking care of critical care patients to the present day. Furthermore, she has received a research grant and has been actively involved in conducting research studies as a principal investigator. She has given several invited presentations at conferences, and has authored many publications in peer-reviewed journals including New England Journal of Medicine and Nephron as a primary and corresponding author.

Preface

As a clinical pharmacist working and teaching for almost 20 years in the intensive care unit (ICU), I have needed to look to different references for different challenging situations. For example, how does one convert opioid dosing when transitioning from home oral oxycodone to intravenous (IV) hydromorphone or IV morphine to transdermal fentanyl? How do we select an anticonvulsant according to a validated clinical practice guideline for a patient in refractory status epilepticus with multiple drug allergies and interactions? What do we choose for an optimal formulary agent within the class of many similar drugs tailored to an individual patient? What source do we use when we are seeking a novel antibiotic for a multidrug-resistant pathogen for a specific type of infection?

Now more than ever, there is overwhelming medical information available as reference books, articles, and online resources. However, they may not be readily available or may be too extensive and complex to search for answers while tending to a critically ill patient at bedside. In my experience, there is no single reference that meets the needs of a clinician who seeks urgently precise and accurate, evidence-based medical information while treating patients in the acute care setting. This fact compelled me to write a pocket book that provides the most current ICU drug information based on practice guidelines, along with expert opinions readily available at hand.

Each chapter is uniquely designed to provide a brief discussion of the disease state, followed by treatment algorithms and drug tables that compare and contrast vital information including pharmacokinetics, pharmacodynamics, drug interactions, adverse effects, contraindication, and hepatic/renal dosing along with clinical pearls to help clinicians decide on optimal drug therapy at glance without a delay.

This book is divided into six sections containing the major clinical ICU areas of practice. Section I highlights pharmacotherapy in cardiovascular critical care, including acute coronary syndromes, acutely decompensated heart failure, adult advanced cardiac life support, anticoagulation for atrial fibrillation/flutter, and hypertensive crisis. Section II addresses management of endocrine emergencies such as diabetic ketoacidosis, hyperosmolar hyperglycemic state, and adrenal and thyroid dysfunction. In addition, treatment strategies for acute pancreatitis, hepatic failure, and gastrointestinal complications such as fistulas, postoperative ileus/nausea/vomiting, and bleeding are depicted.

Section III presents empiric and definitive antimicrobial therapy for infections involving the brain, lung, bloodstream, abdomen, urinary tract, and skin and soft tissue. Section IV reviews pharmacotherapeutic interventions in neurocritical care, including, but not limited to, acute ischemic stroke, status epilepticus, and intracranial hemorrhage. Section V discusses treatment pathways for pulmonary disorders such as asthma and chronic obstructive pulmonary disease exacerbations and pulmonary hypertension. Section VI examines pharmacologic therapies for acute poisoning, anaphylaxis, drug-induced hyperthermia, rapid sequence intubation, venous thromboembolism, fluids and electrolytes, and pain, agitation/sedation, and delirium.

I hope this book becomes a valuable resource for all entry-level clinicians including physicians, pharmacists, nurses, and other healthcare professionals needing a fundamental drug sourcebook while working in ICU, emergency departments, or acute care settings. Furthermore, it can serve as a quick reference that provides a summary or refresher to experienced clinicians working in the hospital setting.

I thank Dr. Morton J Kern for being a magnificent mentor who inspired and advised me throughout the long journey to completion of this book. In addition, I'd like to acknowledge the following invaluable experts for reviewing the chapters:

Ali K. Ashtiani, MD: Chapters 1–5
Ellis R. Levin, MD: Chapters 6 and 7
Timothy R. Morgan, MD: Chapters 8 and 9
Karen Tan, PharmD: Chapters 10 and 11
An T. Tran, MD: Chapters 13–15
Marius C. Viseroi, MD:
Chapters 12, 16–19, 21–22, and 24
Syeda A. Quadri, MD: Chapters 20 and 23
Morton J Kern, MD: All chapters

Jennifer P. Lee, Pharm.D., BCPS
Department of Pharmacy
VA Long Beach, Long Beach, California

Contents

SECTION 6: MISCELLANEOUS

Cardiovascular Critical Care

1

Acute Coronary Syndromes

This chapter will review the pharmacologic management of acute coronary syndromes (ACS) according to the 2013 American College of Cardiology Foundation/American Heart Association (AHA) ST-Elevation Myocardial Infarction (STEMI) and 2014 AHA/American College of Cardiology Non-ST-Elevation Acute Coronary Syndromes (NSTE-ACS) guidelines.

CLINICAL SIGNS AND SYMPTOMS OF ACS (FIG. 1.1)

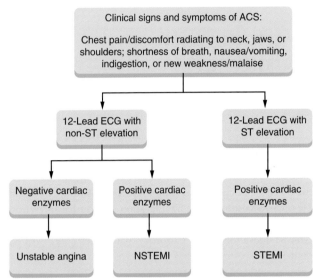

Figure 1.1 Presentation and Diagnosis of Acute Myocardial Infarctions. *Data from Amsterdam EA, Wenger NK, Brindis RG, et al. 2014 AHA/ ACC guideline for the management of patients with non–ST-elevation acute coronary syndromes: executive summary: a report of the American College of Cardiology/American Heart Association Task Force on Practice Guidelines. Circulation. 2014;130:2354–2394. ACS, Acute coronary syndromes; ECG, Electrocardiogram; NSTEMI, Non-ST-elevation myocardial infarction; STEMI, ST-elevation myocardial infarction.*

CAUSES OF TROPONIN ELEVATIONS (BOX 1.1)

Box 1.1 Causes of Troponin Elevations

Acute decompensated heart failure	Early post–cardiac surgery
Acute MI	Heart transplantation
Acute pulmonary embolism	Myocarditis
Aortic stenosis	Pericarditis
Cardiac amyloidosis	Post-PCI
Cardiotoxic chemotherapy	Rhabdomyolysis
Chest compressions	Sepsis
Chest wall trauma	Severe strenuous exercise
Chronic heart failure	Tachyarrhythmia
Direct current cardioversion/defibrillation	Type A dissection

MI, Myocardial infarction; *PCI*, Percutaneous coronary intervention

---

ACUTE MANAGEMENT OF ACS
Goals of Care (Box 1.2)

Box 1.2 Goals of Care

STEMI: REPERFUSION THERAPY	NSTE-ACS: PREVENT TOTAL OCCLUSION OF THE VESSEL
Primary PCI recommended if possible within 90 min of presentation	Revascularization within 24–72 h vs. medical management depending on risk stratification, symptom resolution, and indicators of ongoing myocardial damage/ischemia
If primary PCI impossible within 120 min of medical contact, thrombolytic recommended within 30 min of presentation unless contraindicated	
Surgical revascularization may be indicated	

NSTE-ACS, Non-ST-elevation acute coronary syndromes; *PCI*, Percutaneous coronary intervention; *STEMI*, ST-elevation myocardial infarction
Data from O'Gara PT, Kushner FG, Ascheim DD, et al. ACCF/AHA guideline for the management of ST-elevation myocardial infarction: a report of the American College of Cardiology Foundation/American Heart Association Task Force on Practice Guidelines. Circulation. 2013;127:e362–e425; Amsterdam EA, Wenger NK, Brindis RG, et al. AHA/ACC guideline for the management of patients with non–ST-elevation acute coronary syndromes: executive summary: a report of the American College of Cardiology/American Heart Association Task Force on Practice Guidelines. *Circulation*. 2014;130:2354–2394.

Initial Interventions on Presentation of ACS (Box 1.3)

Box 1.3 Initial Interventions on Presentation of ACS	
Morphine	2–4 mg IV q5min prn chest pain
	Provides analgesia and decreases pain-induced sympathetic tone
	Morphine may induce vasodilation and preload reduction
Oxygen	2–4 L/min by nasal cannula or face mask if hypoxemia (SaO_2 <90%), HF, or dyspnea
	Use cautiously because it may promote coronary vasoconstriction and generate toxic O_2 metabolites
Aspirin	162–325 mg (non-EC) chewed and swallowed immediately, then 81 mg (EC) daily
	Inhibit platelet activation
Nitroglycerin (NTG)	Facilitate coronary vasodilation
	NTG 0.4 mg sublingually or spray q5min ×3. If continuous ischemic pain, HF, or htn, IV NTG 10 mcg/min increased by 5 mcg/min q5min to desired effect (NTE 200 mcg/min)
	Avoid NTG if:
	• SBP <90 mm Hg or SBP ≤30 mm Hg below baseline
	• Severe bradycardia with HR ≤50
	• HR ≥100 in the absence of symptomatic HF, or RV infarction
	• Oral phosphodiesterase inhibitor within the past 24–48 h
β-Blockers	Metoprolol 5 mg IV q5min up to ×3 then 25–50 mg PO q6–12h, transitioned to metoprolol tartrate BID or metoprolol succinate daily
	Decreases risk of ventricular arrhythmias and sudden cardiac death post-MI
	Improves oxygen flow through the coronary arteries
	Initiate within first 24 h of ACS except for:
	• Signs of HF or low-output state
	• Increased risk of cardiogenic shock (SBP <120, HR >110 or <60, age >70)
	• Other CI to β-blockade (i.e., active asthma, reactive airway disease, heart block)

Box 1.3 Initial Interventions on Presentation of ACS—cont'd

Acronym	**M**orphine
MONA ±	**O**xygen
β-Blockers	**N**itroglycerin
	Aspirin
	β-Blocker

ACS, Acute coronary syndromes; *BID*, Twice daily; *CI*, Contraindication; *EC*, Enteric coated; *HF*, Heart failure; *HR*, Heart rate; *htn*, Hypertension; *MI*, Myocardial infarction; *NTE*, Not to exceed; *PO*, Orally; *RV*, Right ventricular; *SBP*, Systolic blood pressure

Data from Amsterdam EA, Wenger NK, Brindis RG, et al. 2014 AHA/ACC guideline for the management of patients with non–ST-elevation acute coronary syndromes: executive summary: a report of the American College of Cardiology/American Heart Association Task Force on Practice Guidelines. *Circulation*. 2014;130:2354–2394.

Additional Intervention in ACS
Management of NSTE-ACS (Fig. 1.2)

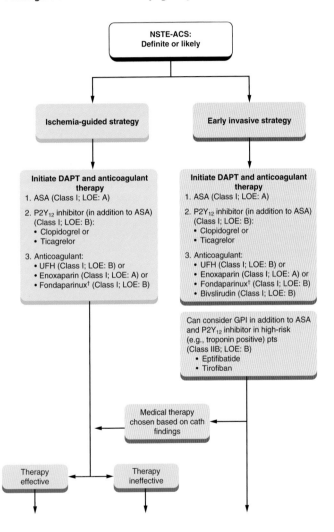

NSTE-ACS:
Definite or likely

Ischemia-guided strategy

Early invasive strategy

Initiate DAPT and anticoagulant therapy
1. ASA (Class I; LOE: A)
2. P2Y₁₂ inhibitor (in addition to ASA) (Class I; LOE: B):
   • Clopidogrel or
   • Ticagrelor
3. Anticoagulant:
   • UFH (Class I; LOE: B) or
   • Enoxaparin (Class I; LOE: A) or
   • Fondaparinux† (Class I; LOE: B)

Initiate DAPT and anticoagulant therapy
1. ASA (Class I; LOE: A)
2. P2Y₁₂ inhibitor (in addition to ASA) (Class I; LOE: B):
   • Clopidogrel or
   • Ticagrelor
3. Anticoagulant:
   • UFH (Class I; LOE: B) or
   • Enoxaparin (Class I; LOE: A) or
   • Fondaparinux† (Class I; LOE: B)
   • Bivslirudin (Class I; LOE: B)

Can consider GPI in addition to ASA and P2Y₁₂ inhibitor in high-risk (e.g., troponin positive) pts (Class IIB; LOE: B)
   • Eptifibatide
   • Tirofiban

Medical therapy chosen based on cath findings

Therapy effective

Therapy ineffective

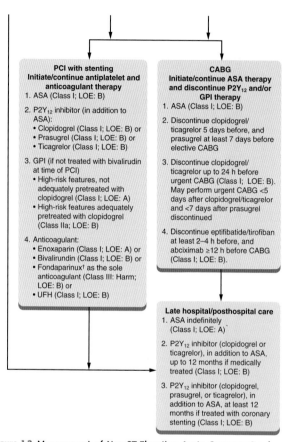

PCI with stenting
Initiate/continue antiplatelet and
anticoagulant therapy
1. ASA (Class I; LOE: B)

2. P2Y₁₂ inhibitor (in addition to
   ASA):
   • Clopidogrel (Class I; LOE: B) or
   • Prasugrel (Class I; LOE: B) or
   • Ticagrelor (Class I; LOE: B)

3. GPI (if not treated with bivalirudin
   at time of PCI)
   • High-risk features, not
     adequately pretreated with
     clopidogrel (Class I; LOE: A)
   • High-risk features adequately
     pretreated with clopidogrel
     (Class IIa; LOE: B)

4. Anticoagulant:
   • Enoxaparin (Class I; LOE: A) or
   • Bivalirudin (Class I; LOE: B) or
   • Fondaparinux† as the sole
     anticoagulant (Class III: Harm;
     LOE: B) or
   • UFH (Class I; LOE: B)

CABG
Initiate/continue ASA therapy
and discontinue P2Y₁₂ and/or
GPI therapy
1. ASA (Class I; LOE: B)

2. Discontinue clopidogrel/
   ticagrelor 5 days before, and
   prasugrel at least 7 days before
   elective CABG

3. Discontinue clopidogrel/
   ticagrelor up to 24 h before
   urgent CABG (Class I; LOE: B).
   May perform urgent CABG <5
   days after clopidogrel/ticagrelor
   and <7 days after prasugrel
   discontinued

4. Discontinue eptifibatide/tirofiban
   at least 2–4 h before, and
   abciximab ≥12 h before CABG
   (Class I; LOE: B).

Late hospital/posthospital care
1. ASA indefinitely
   (Class I; LOE: A)

2. P2Y₁₂ inhibitor (clopidogrel or
   ticagrelor), in addition to ASA,
   up to 12 months if medically
   treated (Class I; LOE: B)

3. P2Y₁₂ inhibitor (clopidogrel,
   prasugrel, or ticagrelor), in
   addition to ASA, at least 12
   months if treated with coronary
   stenting (Class I; LOE: B)

Figure 1.2 Management of Non-ST-Elevation Acute Coronary Syndrome.
*From Amsterdam EA, Wenger NK, Brindis RG, et al. 2014 AHA/ACC guideline
for the management of patients with non–ST-elevation acute coronary
syndromes: executive summary: a report of the American College of
Cardiology/American Heart Association Task Force on Practice Guidelines.
Circulation. 2014;130:2354–2394.* †Additional UFH or bivalirudin should
be given at the time of PCI because of the risk of catheter thrombosis.
ASA, Aspirin; *CABG,* Coronary artery bypass graft; *DAPT,* Dual antiplatelet
therapy; *GPI,* Glycoprotein IIb/IIIa inhibitor; *NSTE-ACS,* Non-ST-elevation
acute coronary syndromes; *PCI,* Percutaneous coronary intervention;
UFH, Unfractionated heparin. *Class I,* Strong recommendation; *Class IIa,*
Reasonable recommendation; *Class IIb,* May be considered; *Class III,* No befit;
LOE: A, Multiple populations evaluated; *LOE: B,* Limited populations evaluated.

Oral Antiplatelets (Table 1.1)

Table 1.1 Oral Antiplatelet Therapy

DRUG	ASPIRIN	CLOPIDOGREL	PRASUGREL	TICAGRELOR
Mechanism of action	Inhibits thromboxane A$_2$-mediated platelet activation	Inhibits ADP-mediated platelet activation at P2Y$_{12}$ receptor		
Loading dose	162–325 mg	600 mg[a]	60 mg	180 mg
Maintenance dose	81 mg daily	75 mg daily	10 mg daily[b]	90 mg BID
Prodrug	No	Yes	Yes	No
Reversible platelet binding	No	No	No	Yes
Onset	30 min	2–6 h	30 min	30 min
Platelet inhibition	10–20%	30–40%	60–70%	60–70%
Hold before CABG	Do not hold	5 days	7 days	5 days

| Comments | Non-EC formulation for loading then EC formulation for maintenance | Pharmacogenomic variability (CYP2C19) in response | CI: history of stroke/TIA; bleeding risk Caution: age ≥75 yr, weight <60 kg | Avoid concomitant ASA >100 mg daily (lack of efficacy) |

Notes:

- Aspirin plus P2Y$_{12}$ for up to 12 months for patients treated initially with an invasive or ischemia-guided strategy
- Aspirin plus P2Y$_{12}$ for at least 12 months for patients treated with coronary stents

ADP, Adenosine diphosphate; ASA, Aspirin; BID, Twice daily; CABG, Coronary artery bypass grafting; CI, Contraindication; CYP, Cytochrome P450 enzymes; EC, Enteric coated; TIA, Transient ischemic attack

[a]300 mg loading for ≤75 yr and no loading for >75 yr receiving fibrinolytic

[b]Patients with weight <60 kg should receive 5 mg daily

Data from O'Gara PT, Kushner FG, Ascheim DD, et al. 2013 ACCF/AHA guideline for the management of ST-elevation myocardial infarction: a report of the American College of Cardiology Foundation/American Heart Association Task Force on Practice Guidelines. Circulation. 2013;127:e362–e425; Amsterdam EA, Wenger NK, Brindis RG, et al. 2014 AHA/ACC guideline for the management of patients with non–ST-elevation acute coronary syndromes: executive summary: a report of the American College of Cardiology/American Heart Association Task Force on Practice Guidelines. Circulation. 2014;130:2354–2394; Levine GN, Bates ER, Blankenship JC, et al. 2011 ACCF/AHA/SCAI guideline for percutaneous coronary intervention: a report of the American College of Cardiology Foundation/American Heart Association Task Force on Practice Guidelines and the Society for Cardiovascular Angiography and Interventions. J Am Coll Cardiol. 2011;58:e44–e122; Wijeyeratne YD, Heptinstall S. Anti-platelet therapy: ADP receptor antagonists. Br J Clin Pharmacol. 2011;4:647–657.

Parenteral Antithrombotics for Percutaneous Coronary Intervention (Table 1.2)

Table 1.2 Parenteral Antithrombotics for PCI

DRUG	LD (IV)	MD (IV)	RETURN OF PLT FUNCTION AFTER DC	ELIMINATION	DIALYZABLE
Indirect Thrombin Inhibitor					
UFH	With GP IIb/IIIa inhibitor: 50–70 units/kg Without GP IIb/IIIa inhibitor: 70–100 units/kg	Rebolus to maintain goal ACT during procedure With GP IIb/IIIa inhibitor: 200–250 s Without GP IIb/IIIa inhibitor: 250–300 s	—	Hepatic and RES	No
Direct Thrombin Inhibitor					
Bivalirudin (Angiomax)	0.75 mg/kg Additional 0.3 mg/kg if needed	1.75 mg/kg/h CrCl <30: 1 mg/kg/h With or without UFH	1 h	80% plasma proteolysis 20% renal	Partial
GP IIa/IIIa Inhibitors					
Abciximab (ReoPro) Not in U.S.	0.25 mg/kg	0.125 mcg/kg/min Max: 10 mcg/min	24–72 h; Up to 7 days	RES	No

Eptifibatide (Integrilin)	180 mcg/kg q10min ×2	2 mcg/kg/min CrCl <50: 1 mcg/kg/min HD: avoid	4–8 h	50% renal	Yes
Tirofiban (Aggrastat)	25 mcg/kg	0.15 mcg/kg/min CrCl <60: 0.075 mcg/kg/min	4–8 h	65% renal	Yes
Direct P2Y$_{12}$ Platelet Receptor Inhibitor					
Cangrelor (Kengreal)	30 mcg/kg	4 mcg/kg/min	1 h	Plasma dephos-phorylation	N/A

ACT, Activated clotting time; CrCl, Creatinine clearance; DC, Discontinuation; GP, Glycoprotein; HD, Hemodialysis; IV, Intravenously; LD, Loading dose; MD, Maintenance dose; N/A, Not applicable; PCI, Percutaneous coronary intervention; PLT, Platelet; RES, Reticuloendothelial system; UFH, Unfractionated heparin

Data from O'Gara PT, Kushner FG, Ascheim DD, et al. 2013 ACCF/AHA guideline for the management of ST-elevation myocardial infarction: a report of the American College of Cardiology Foundation/American Heart Association Task Force on Practice Guidelines. *Circulation*. 2013;127:e362–e425; Amsterdam EA, Wenger NK, Brindis RG, et al. 2014 AHA/ACC guideline for the management of patients with non–ST-elevation acute coronary syndromes: executive summary: a report of the American College of Cardiology/American Heart Association Task Force on Practice Guidelines. *Circulation*. 2014;130:2354–2394; Wijeyeratne YD, Heptinstall S. Anti-platelet therapy: ADP receptor antagonists. *Br J Clin Pharmacol*. 2011;4:647–657.

Thrombolytics (Table 1.3)

Table 1.3 Thrombolytic Therapy for STEMI

DRUG	STANDARD DOSING (IV)	PD/PK	COMMENT
Alteplase	15 mg bolus over 1–2 min, then 0.75 mg/kg (NTE 50 mg) over 30 min, then 0.5 mg/kg (NTE 35 mg) over 60 min Maximum: 100 mg over 90 min	Hepatic metabolism >50% cleared within 5 min after infusion completed, 80% cleared within 10 min	Original and slow-acting thrombolytic but clinical outcomes are no different
Tenecteplase	<60 kg: 30 mg 60–69 kg: 35 mg 70–79 kg: 40 mg 80–89 kg: 45 mg ≥90 kg: 50 mg All doses given as bolus over 5–10 s	Hepatic metabolism Half-life elimination: Initial: 20–24 min Terminal: 90–130 min	Fast-acting thrombolytic but clinical outcomes are no different

Notes:
- Thrombolytic should be administered within 30 min of hospital arrival
- Administer concurrent aspirin, clopidogrel, and anticoagulant (UFH, enoxaparin, or fondaparinux)
- UFH: 60 units/kg IV bolus, then 12 units/kg/h titrated to target aPTT 1.5–2 times control for 48 h or until revascularization
- Enoxaparin
  - STEMI and <75 yr: 30 mg IV ×1 then in 15 min 1 mg/kg subq q12h (max 100 mg for first two doses)
  - STEMI and ≥75 yr: 0.75 mg/kg subq q12h (max 75 mg for first two doses)
  - Up to 8 days or until revascularization
  - CrCl <30: same bolus as above then maintenance dose q24h
- Fondaparinux: 2.5 mg IV ×1 then 2.5 mg subq daily starting the following day; contraindicated in CrCl <30

aPTT, Activated partial thromboplastin time; *CrCl*, Creatinine clearance; *IV*, Intravenously; *NTE*, Not to exceed; *PD/PK*, Pharmacodynamics/pharmacokinetics; *STEMI*, ST-elevation myocardial infarction; *subq*, subcutaneously; *UFH*, Unfractionated heparin

Contraindications (Table 1.4)

Table 1.4 Contraindications to Thrombolytic Therapy

ABSOLUTE CONTRAINDICATIONS	RELATIVE CONTRAINDICATIONS
Active bleeding excluding menses	Systolic BP >180 mm Hg or diastolic BP >110 mm Hg
Intracranial neoplasm	Active bleeding in past 4 weeks
Arteriovenous malformation or aneurysm	Non-compressible vascular punctures
Suspected aortic dissection	Major surgery in past 3 weeks
Ischemic stroke within 3 months	Traumatic or prolonged (>10 min) cardiopulmonary resuscitation
Prior intracranial hemorrhage	
Significant closed head or facial trauma within 3 months	Ischemic stroke >3 months ago
Intracranial/intraspinal surgery/trauma within 2 months	Dementia
	Active peptic ulcer disease
	Pregnancy
Bleeding diathesis	Ongoing therapy with warfarin

Data from O'Gara PT, Kushner FG, Ascheim DD, et al. 2013 ACCF/AHA guideline for the management of ST-elevation myocardial infarction: a report of the American College of Cardiology Foundation/American Heart Association Task Force on Practice Guidelines. *Circulation.* 2013;127:e362–e425.

Medical Therapies for Stabilized ACS (Table 1.5)

Table 1.5 Routine Medical Therapies for Stabilized ACS

CLASS	INDICATIONS	ORAL DRUG REGIMEN (TARGET DOSE)	AVOID/CAUTION
β-Blockers	All patients without CI	Metoprolol tartrate 25–50 mg q6–12h, transitioned to BID of metoprolol tartrate or daily of metoprolol succinate[a] (200 mg/day) Carvedilol 6.25 mg BID (25 mg BID) Bisoprolol 1.25 mg daily (10 mg daily)	Signs of HF, low output state Increased risk of cardiogenic shock Prolonged first-degree or high-grade AV block Reactive airway disease
ACEI	All patients with anterior infarction, post-MI LV systolic dysfunction (EF ≤40%), or HF All patients without CI	Lisinopril 2.5–5 mg daily (10 mg daily) Captopril 6.25–12.5 mg TID (25–50 mg TID) Ramipril 2.5 mg BID (5 mg BID) Trandolapril 0.5 mg daily (4 mg daily)	Hypotension Renal failure Hyperkalemia
ARB	For patients intolerant of ACEI	Valsartan 20 mg BID (160 mg BID)	Hypotension Renal failure Hyperkalemia
Statins	All patients without CI	Atorvastatin 80 mg daily	DDI: CYP3A4, fibrates Monitor for myopathy, hepatic toxicity

ACS, Acute coronary syndrome; ACEI, Angiotensin converting enzyme inhibitor; ARB, Angiotensin receptor blocker; AV, Atrioventricular; BID, Twice daily; CI, contraindication; CYP, cytochrome P450 enzymes; DDI, Drug-drug interaction; EF, Ejection fraction; HF, Heart failure; LV, Left ventricle; MI, Myocardial infarction; TID, Three times daily.

[a]Succinate form rather than tartrate recommended if concomitant non-ST-elevation myocardial infarction, stable HF, or reduced systolic function

Data from O'Gara PT, Kushner FG, Ascheim DD, et al. 2013 ACCF/AHA guideline for the management of ST-elevation myocardial infarction: a report of the American College of Cardiology Foundation/American Heart Association Task Force on Practice Guidelines. *Circulation.* 2013;127:e362–e425.

References

1. O'Gara PT, Kushner FG, Ascheim DD, et al. ACCF/AHA guideline for the management of ST-elevation myocardial infarction: a report of the American College of Cardiology Foundation/American Heart Association Task Force on Practice Guidelines. *Circulation*. 2013;127:e362–e425.

2. Amsterdam EA, Wenger NK, Brindis RG, et al. AHA/ACC guideline for the management of patients with non–ST-elevation acute coronary syndromes: executive summary: a report of the American College of Cardiology/American Heart Association Task Force on Practice Guidelines. *Circulation*. 2014;130:2354–2394.

3. Levine GN, Bates ER, Blankenship JC, et al. ACCF/AHA/SCAI guideline for percutaneous coronary intervention: a report of the American College of Cardiology Foundation/American Heart Association Task Force on Practice Guidelines and the Society for Cardiovascular Angiography and Interventions. *J Am Coll Cardiol*. 2011;58:e44–e122.

4. Wijeyeratne YD, Heptinstall S. Anti-platelet therapy: ADP receptor antagonists. *Br J Clin Pharmacol*. 2011;4:647–657.

2

Acutely Decompensated Heart Failure (ADHF)

This chapter will review the pharmacologic management of heart failure (HF) according to the American College of Cardiology Foundation/American Heart Association/Heart Failure Society of America Practice Guidelines.

DEFINITIONS

- ADHF: new or worsening signs and symptoms of HF, characterized by acute dyspnea associated with elevated intra-cardiac filling pressures with or without pulmonary edema.
- HF with reduced ejection fraction (HFrEF): ejection fraction (EF) ≤40%.
- HF with preserved EF (HFpEF): EF ≥50%.
- HFpEF, borderline: EF 41–49%.
- Stages of HF
  - Stage A: normal cardiac function/morphology with increased risk of HF
  - Stage B: abnormal cardiac function/morphology without symptoms of HF
  - Stage C: symptomatic HF
  - Stage D: end-stage HF
- New York Heart Association (NYHA) functional classification:
  - NYHA I: no limitation of physical activity
  - NYHA II: slight limitation of physical activity
  - NYHA III: marked limitation of physical activity
  - NYHA IV: symptoms at rest

PRECIPITATING FACTORS

- Nonadherence with diet
- Worsening renal failure
- Uncontrolled hypertension
- Infection
- Pulmonary embolism
- Myocardial ischemia, arrhythmias
- Hyperthyroidism/hypothyroidism
- Drugs (Table 2.1)

Table 2.1 Critical Care Drugs That Can Promote Heart Failure

THERAPEUTIC CLASS AND DRUG	POSSIBLE MECHANISM
Analgesics	
NSAIDs (i.e., Ketorolac) COX-2 inhibitors (i.e., Celocoxib)	Prostaglandin inhibition resulting in sodium/water retention and blunted diuretic response
Anesthesia Medications	
Desflurane, isoflurane, sevoflurane	Myocardial depression and peripheral vasodilation
Dexmedetomidine	α-Receptor agonist
Etomidate	Adrenal suppression
Ketamine	Negative inotrope
Propofol	Negative inotrope and vasodilation
Calcium Channel Blockers	
Diltiazem, verapamil, nifedipine	Negative inotrope
Anti-Infective Medications	
Itraconazole	Negative inotrope
Amphotericin	Unknown
Ampicillin/sulbactam	High sodium content
Azithromycin (injection)	"
Metronidazole (injection)	"
Nafcillin	"
Oxacillin	"
Piperacillin/tazobactam	"
Ticarcillin/clavulanate potassium	"

Continued

Table 2.1 Critical Care Drugs That Can Promote Heart
Failure—cont'd

THERAPEUTIC CLASS AND DRUG	POSSIBLE MECHANISM
Pulmonary Medications	
Albuterol	Decreased β-receptor responsiveness with chronic use
Epoprostenol	Unknown
Bosentan	"
Miscellaneous	
Polyethylene glycol	High sodium content in formulation
Sodium phosphates enema	
Sodium polystyrene sulfonate	"

COX-2, Cyclooxygenase-2; *NSAIDs*, Nonsteroidal antiinflammatory drugs
Data from Page RL II, O'Bryant CL, Chen D, et al. Drugs that may cause or exacerbate heart failure:
a scientific statement from the American Heart Association. *Circulation.* 2016;134:e32–e69.

PHARMACOLOGIC MANAGEMENT

Vasodilator

For treatment of normotensive or hypertensive HF; lacks
unwanted cardiac stimulation (Table 2.2)

Inodilator

For systolic dysfunction when vasodilator therapy is not
tolerated due to hypotension (Table 2.3)

Diuretic Therapy

Only if hypervolemia or elevated pulmonary artery wedge
pressure (>20 mm Hg) despite vasodilator or inodilator therapy (Tables 2.4 and 2.5). Must be combined with vasodilator
or inodilator.

Vasopressin Receptor Antagonist

- Tolvaptan: most studied
- Adjunct to diuretics and other standard therapies for
  ADHF
- Short-term use (tolvaptan should not be used >30 days)
  for volume overload with persistent severe hyponatremia

Table 2.2 Continuous-Infusion Vasodilator Therapy

DRUG	STANDARD DOSING (IV)	COMMENT
Nitroglycerin (NTG)	Start at 5 mcg/min Titrate by 5 mcg/min q5min to achieve desired hemodynamic effect Max 200 mcg/min	Preferred vasodilator, especially in patients with CAD Greater venous than arterial vasodilation Tachyphylaxis can occur after 16–24 h of continuous NTG administration ADR: methemoglobinemia (rare) CI: Phosphodiesterase-5 enzyme inhibitors such as sildenafil
Nitroprusside	Start at 5 mcg/min Titrate by 5 mcg/min q5min to achieve desired hemodynamic effect Max dose: 400 mcg/min Max duration: 72 h	Preferred in severe hypertension, acute mitral regurgitation, or acute aortic regurgitation Balanced arterial and venous dilation Monitor for cyanide toxicity Not recommended in renal/hepatic insufficiency CI: myocardial ischemia
Nesiritide (no longer available in U.S.)	Start with a bolus 2 mcg/kg, then 0.01 mcg/kg/min Titrate by 0.005 mcg/kg/min q3h Max 0.03 mcg/kg/min	Recombinant human B-type natriuretic peptide with same natriuretic and vasodilator effects as endogenous BNP Balanced arterial and venous dilation

ADR, Adverse drug reaction; *BNP*, Brain natriuretic peptide; *CAD*, Coronary artery disease; *CI*, Contraindication; *IV*, Intravenously
Data from Yancy CW, Jessup M, Bozkurt B, et al. 2013 ACCF/AHA guideline for the management of heart failure: executive summary: a report of the American College of Cardiology Foundation/American Heart Association Task Force on Practice Guidelines. *Circulation.* 2013;128:1810–1852.

Table 2.3 Continuous-Infusion Inodilator Therapy

DRUG	STANDARD DOSING (IV)	COMMENT
Dobutamine	Start at 2.5 mcg/kg/min Titrate by 2.5 mcg/kg/min if needed Range: 5–20 mcg/kg/min	Potent β_1-receptor agonist: positive inotropic effects Weak $\beta_2 \geq \alpha_1$ receptor agonist: vasodilation in addition to inotropic and chronotropic effects ADR: tachycardia, increase in myocardial O_2 consumption, increase/decrease in blood pressure Least preferred due to deleterious effects of adrenergic stimulation
Dopamine	5–10 mcg/kg/min	Consider in addition to loop diuretic therapy to improve diuresis Dose-related receptor activity: 2–5 mcg/kg/min: dopamine receptor 5–10 mcg/kg/min: β_1-receptor >10 mcg/kg/min: α_1-receptor
Levosimendan (not available in U.S.)	Bolus 12 mcg/kg over 10 min, then 0.1 mcg/kg/min Max dose: 0.2 mcg/kg/min Max duration: 24 h	Increases cardiac contractility by sensitizing cardiac myofilaments to calcium Promotes vasodilation by facilitating potassium influx into vascular smooth muscle Preferred agent especially in myocardial ischemia or infarction
Milrinone	Bolus 50 mcg/kg over 10 min, then 0.375–0.75 mcg/kg/min CrCl 50: 0.43 mcg/kg/min CrCl 40: 0.38 mcg/kg/min CrCl 30: 0.33 mcg/kg/min CrCl 20: 0.28 mcg/kg/min CrCl 10: 0.23 mcg/kg/min CrCl 5: 0.2 mcg/kg/min	Phosphodiesterase inhibitor: enhances myocardial contractility and relaxation Less tachycardia than dobutamine but similar risk of ventricular arrhythmias Preferred over dobutamine if recent administration of β-blocker or concomitant pulmonary hypertension Slower onset and longer half-life than dobutamine

ADR, Adverse drug reaction; CrCl, Creatinine clearance

Data from Yancy CW, Jessup M, Bozkurt B, et al. 2013 ACCF/AHA guideline for the management of heart failure: executive summary: a report of the American College of Cardiology Foundation/American Heart Association Task Force on Practice Guidelines. *Circulation.* 2013;128:1810–1852.

Table 2.4 Diuretic Therapy in Diuretic Naïve and Normal Renal Function

DRUG	INITIAL DOSE (IV)	USUAL MAXIMUM DOSE (IV)	ORAL BIOAVAIL-ABILITY	ORAL DOSE EQUIVA-LENCY
Furosemide	20–40 mg	200 mg	50%	40 mg
Bumetanide	1 mg	8 mg	80%	1 mg
Torsemide	10–20 mg	100 mg	80%	20 mg

Notes:
- If minimal response to the initial dose, double the dose q2h as needed up to the maximum recommended dose.
- Onset of diuresis 30 min and peak of diuresis 1–2 h after IV diuretic administration

IV, Intravenous

Data from Yancy CW, Jessup M, Bozkurt B, et al. 2013 ACCF/AHA guideline for the management of heart failure: executive summary: a report of the American College of Cardiology Foundation/American Heart Association Task Force on Practice Guidelines. *Circulation.* 2013;128:1810–1852.

Table 2.5 Diuretic Therapy in Diuretic Resistance or Renal Insufficiency

	FUROSEMIDE		METOLAZONE
PRIOR DAILY ORAL DOSE	IV BOLUS	CONTINUOUS INFUSION	ORAL DOSE
≤80 mg	40 mg	5 mg/h	—
81–160 mg	80 mg	10 mg/h	5 mg daily
161–240 mg	80 mg	20 mg/h	5 mg BID
>240 mg	80 mg	30 mg/h	5 mg BID

Notes:
- Goal diuresis is 3–5 liters of urine per day until clinical euvolemia is reached
- Hydrochlorothiazide 50 mg BID or chlorthalidone 50 mg daily may be substituted for metolazone

BID, Two times daily; *IV,* Intravenously.

From Ellison DH, Felker GM. Diuretic treatment in heart failure. *N Engl J Med.* 2017;377:1964–1975.

(Na ≤120 mEq/L; correct for hyperglycemia if appropriate) despite water restriction and maximal medical therapy
- Caution: hepatotoxicity
- Use controversial due to unknown long-term safety

Guideline-Directed Medical Therapy for Stage C HF*r*EF

- Treatment algorithm (Fig. 2.1)
- Pharmacological management (Table 2.6)

Venous Thromboembolism Prophylaxis Unless Contraindicated (see Table 24.2)

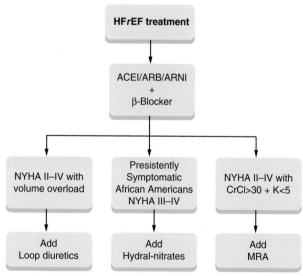

Figure 2.1 Guideline-Directed Medical Therapy for HfrEF. *Data from Yancy CW, Jessup M, Bozkurt B, et al. 2013 ACCF/AHA guideline for the management of heart failure: executive summary: a report of the American College of Cardiology Foundation/American Heart Association Task Force on Practice Guidelines. Circulation. 2013;128:1810–1852. ACEI, Angiotensin-converting enzyme inhibitor; ARB, Angiotensin-receptor blocker; ARNI, Angiotensin receptor-neprilysin inhibitor; CrCl, Creatinine clearance; HFrEF, Heart failure with reduced ejection fraction; Hydral-Nitrates, Hydralazine and isosorbide dinitrate; K, Potassium; MRA, Mineralocorticoid receptor antagonists; NYHA, New York Heart Association.*

Table 2.6 Long-Term Therapy for Systolic Dysfunction

DRUG	INITIAL DOSE (PO)	TARGET DOSE (PO)	COMMENTS
Angiotensin-Converting Enzyme Inhibitors (ACEIs)			
Captopril	6.25 mg TID	50 mg TID	Titrate dose q1–2 weeks
Enalapril (Vasotec)	2.5 mg BID	10–20 mg BID	Caution: hypotension, hyponatremia, diabetes, volume depletion, renal disease, potassium >5 mEq (mmol)/L, advanced age
Fosinopril	5–10 mg daily	40 mg daily	
Lisinopril (Prinivil, Zestril)	2.5–5 mg daily	20–40 mg daily	
Perindopril (Aceon)	2 mg daily	8–16 mg daily	
Quinapril (Accupril)	5 mg BID	20 mg BID	
Ramipril (Altace)	1.25–2.5 mg daily	10 mg daily	
Trandolapril (Mavik)	1 mg daily	4 mg daily	
Angiotensin II Receptor Blockers (ARBs)			
Candesartan (Atacand)	4–8 mg daily	32 mg daily	For patients intolerant to ACEI
Losartan (Cozaar)	25–50 mg daily	50–150 mg daily	Titration and caution as per ACEIs above
Valsartan (Diovan)	20–40 mg daily	160 mg BID	
Sacubitril/valsartan (Entresto)	24/26–49/51 mg BID	97/103 mg BID	Sacubitril in Entresto is a neprilysin inhibitor

Continued

Table 2.6 Long-Term Therapy for Systolic Dysfunction.—cont'd

DRUG	INITIAL DOSE (PO)	TARGET DOSE (PO)	COMMENTS
β-Blockers			
Bisoprolol	1.25 mg daily	10 mg daily	Bisoprolol and metoprolol: β_1 selective
Carvedilol (Coreg)	3.125 mg BID	50 mg BID	Carvedilol: blocks β_1, β_2, and α_1 receptors
Carvedilol extended-release (Coreg CR)	10 mg daily	80 mg daily	Do not up-titrate dose until ADR resolved
Metoprolol succinate extended-release (Toprol-XL)	12.5–25 mg daily	200 mg daily	Metoprolol tartrate immediate-release has no indication for heart failure
Mineralocorticoid Receptor Antagonists (MRAs)			
Eplerenone (Inspra)	25 mg daily CrCl 30–49: 25 mg every other day	50 mg daily CrCl 30–49 or with moderate CYP3A4 inhibitors: 25 mg daily	Do not start if SCr ≥2.5 mg/dL in men or ≥2 mg/dL in women, CrCl ≤30, or potassium ≥5 mEq/L Discontinue if potassium >5.5 mEq/L Increase to target dose after 4 weeks if potassium ≤5 mEq/L
Spironolactone (Aldactone)	12.5–25 mg daily CrCl 30–49: 12.5 mg daily or every other day	25 mg daily or BID CrCl 30–49: 12.5–25 mg daily	

Vasodilators

Hydralazine	25–50 mg TID–QID	100 mg TID	Isosorbide dinitrate 20 mg + hydralazine 37.5 mg (BiDil) Initial dose: one tablet TID Target dose: two tablets TID
Isosorbide dinitrate (Isordil)	20–30 mg TID–QID	40 mg TID	

Notes:

- ACEI/ARB can usually be started 24–48 h after presentation, once patient is hemodynamically stable
- Recommend starting a β-blocker after optimization of volume status and discontinuation of intravenous diuretics, vasodilators, and inotropic agents
- Recommend angiotensin receptor-neprilysin inhibitor (ARNI) for patients who have tolerated high doses of ACEI/ARB (≥Enalapril 10 mg BID equivalent)
- Criteria for initiating the ARNI Sacubitril/valsartan: elevated natriuretic peptide level, SBP ≥100, GFR ≥30, and no history of angioedema
- ACEI, ARB, or ARNI, β-blocker, and MRA reduce morbidity and mortality
- Isosorbide mononitrate extended-release (30–120 mg daily) may substitute isosorbide dinitrate for better adherence
- Ivabradin (Corlanor)
  - A new agent that selectively inhibits the I_f current in the sinoatrial node leading to decrease in heart rate
  - Reduces HF hospitalization for patients with stable, symptomatic (NYHA II–III) chronic HF with EF ≤35% who are on a maximally tolerated β-blocker (or contraindication to β-blocker) and in sinus rhythm with resting heart rate ≥70
  - Dose: 2.5–7.5 mg twice daily

ADR, Adverse drug reaction; BID, Two times daily; CrCl, Creatinine clearance; CYP, Cytochrome P450 enzymes; EF, Ejection fraction; GFR, Glomerular filtration rate; HF, Heart failure; NYHA, New York Heart Association; PO, Orally; QID, Four times daily; SBP, Systolic blood pressure; TID, Three times daily

Drugs without brand names are denoted by generic name only

Data from Yancy CW, Jessup M, Bozkurt B, et al. 2013 ACCF/AHA guideline for the management of heart failure: executive summary: a report of the American College of Cardiology Foundation/American Heart Association Task Force on Practice Guidelines. Circulation. 2013;128:1810–1852.

References

1. Page RL II, O'Bryant CL, Chen D, et al. Drugs that may cause or exacerbate heart failure: a scientific statement from the American Heart Association. *Circulation.* 2016;134:e32–e69.
2. Yancy CW, Jessup M, Bozkurt B, et al. 2013 ACCF/AHA guideline for the management of heart failure: executive summary: a report of the American College of Cardiology Foundation/American Heart Association Task Force on Practice Guidelines. *Circulation.* 2013;128:1810–1852.
3. Ellison DH, Felker GM. Diuretic treatment in heart failure. *N Engl J Med.* 2017;377:1964–1975.

3

Adult Advanced Cardiovascular Life Support

This chapter will review the current recommendations from the American Heart Association Guidelines for Cardiopulmonary Resuscitation and Emergency Cardiovascular Care.

ASYSTOLE/PULSELESS ELECTRICAL ACTIVITY
- Algorithm (Fig. 3.1)
- Pharmacologic management (Table 3.1)

VENTRICULAR FIBRILLATION/PULSELESS VENTRICULAR TACHYCARDIA
- Algorithm (Fig. 3.2)
- Pharmacologic management (see Table 3.1)

BRADYCARDIA WITH PULSE
- Algorithm (Fig. 3.3)
- Pharmacologic management (see Table 3.1)

TACHYCARDIA WITH PULSE
- Algorithm (Fig. 3.4)
- Pharmacologic management (see Table 3.1)

POST-CARDIAC ARREST CARE
- Algorithm (Fig. 3.5)
- Pharmacologic management (Table 3.2)

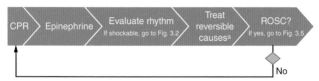

Figure 3.1 Algorithm for Asystole and PEA. *Data from Panchal AR, Berg KM, Kudenchuk PJ, et al. 2018 American Heart Association focused update on advanced cardiovascular life support use of antiarrhythmic drugs during and immediately after cardiac arrest. Circulation. 2018;138:e740–e749.* CPR, Cardiopulmonary resuscitation; *PEA*, Pulseless electrical activity; ROSC, Return of spontaneous circulation. [a]5 H's, hypovolemia, hypoxia, hydrogen ion (acidosis), hypo-/hyperkalemia, and hypothermia. 5 T's, tension pneumothorax, tamponade (cardiac), toxins, thrombosis (pulmonary), and thrombosis (coronary).

TARGETED TEMPERATURE MANAGEMENT (TTM) OR THERAPEUTIC HYPOTHERMIA (TH)[4]

- Fever in the post–cardiac arrest patient not treated with TTM is associated with poor outcome.
- Should be considered for any comatose patient with ROSC after cardiac arrest.
- Target temperature 32–36°C for at least 24 h. Active rewarming not recommended.
- Complications of TTM and management (Table 3.3).

Table 3.1 Antiarrhythmic Drugs for ACLS

DRUG	STANDARD DOSING	MOA	COMMENTS
Asystole/PEA and VF/pVT (see Fig. 3.1 and 3.2)			
Epinephrine	IV/IO: 1 mg q3–5min ET: 2–2.5 mg q3–5min (dilute with 5–10 mL of NS or sterile water)	α-Adrenergic agonist vasoconstriction	↑ Coronary and cerebral perfusion pressure during CPR ↑ ROSC; ↑ survival to hospital admission in out-of-hospital arrests
VF/pVT (see Fig. 3.2)			
Amiodarone	IV/IO: First dose: 300 mg Second dose: 150 mg	Na/K/Ca channel and β-receptor antagonist; Class III antiarrhythmic	Administer as push if pulseless For VF/pVT refractory to defibrillation
Lidocaine	IV/IO: First dose: 1–1.5 mg/kg Second dose: 0.5–0.75 mg/kg	Na channel antagonist; Class Ib antiarrhythmic	For VF/pVT refractory to defibrillation Increased risk of toxicities in hepatic dysfunction, HF, and elderly
Magnesium	IV/IO: 1–2 g over 5 min (diluted in 10 mL of 5% dextrose or sterile water)	Stops EAD by inhibiting Ca channel influx	Optimal dosing not established Indicated in Torsades de pointes

Continued

Table 3.1 Antiarrhythmic Drugs for ACLS—cont'd

DRUG	STANDARD DOSING	MOA	COMMENTS
Bradycardia With Pulse (see Fig. 3.3)			
Atropine	IV: 0.5 mg q3–5min Maximum: 3 mg	Blocks acetylcholine at parasympathetic sites in smooth muscle; ↑ cardiac output	First-line for acute symptomatic bradycardia
Dopamine	IV: 2–10 mcg/kg/min	β-Adrenergic agonist with rate-accelerating effect	For bradycardia unresponsive to atropine
Epinephrine	IV: 2–10 mcg/min	β-Adrenergic agonist with rate-accelerating effect	For bradycardia unresponsive to atropine
Tachycardia With Pulse (see Fig. 3.4)			
Adenosine	First dose: 6 mg IV Second dose: 12 mg IV Administer rapidly over 1–2 s Follow each dose with 20 mL NS flush	Slows conduction time and interrupts reentry pathways through the AV node	Drug of choice for re-entrant tachycardias involving the AV node Reduce initial dose to 3 mg if concurrent carbamazepine or dipyridamole, transplanted heart, or central line administration

Drug	Dose	Mechanism	Notes
Amiodarone	IV: 150 mg over 10 min (may repeat) then 1 mg/min ×6 h, followed by 0.5 mg/min ×18 h Max dose: 2.2 g/24 h	Na/K/Ca channel and β-receptor antagonist; Class III antiarrhythmic	Administer as slow infusion if pulse obtained Preferred in AF with HF Can convert AF to sinus rhythm: embolic risk ADR: hypotension, bradycardia, elevated liver enzymes, phlebitis DDI: inhibits digoxin and warfarin metabolism via cytochrome P450
Procainamide	IV: 20–50 mg/min until arrhythmia resolved Maximum: 17 mg/kg Maintenance: 1–4 mg/min	↓ Myocardial excitability and conduction velocity; Class Ia antiarrhythmic	Avoid if prolonged QT or HF
Sotalol	IV: 100 mg over 5 min	β_1 and β_2 receptor antagonist; Class II and III antiarrhythmic	Avoid if prolonged QT
Metoprolol	2.5–5 mg IV over 2 min; repeat q5–10min up to three doses	Cardioselective β_1 receptor antagonists	Preferred in AF associated with hyperadrenergic states (e.g., acute MI, post-cardiac surgery)
Esmolol	IV: 500 mcg/kg then 50 mcg/kg/min; titrate by 25 mcg/kg/min q5min Max: 200 mcg/kg/min	Cardioselective β_1 receptor antagonists	Ultra-short-acting; rapid dose titration Preferred in AF associated with hyperadrenergic states

Continued

Table 3.1 Antiarrhythmic Drugs for ACLS—cont'd

DRUG	STANDARD DOSING	MOA	COMMENTS
Diltiazem	IV: 0.25 mg/kg over 2 min (may repeat bolus with 0.35 mg/kg), then 5–15 mg/h	Ca channel blocker	Possess negative inotropic effects; however, safely used in HF ADR: hypotension, cardiac depression
Verapamil	IV: 0.25–5 mg over 2 min; may repeat q15–30min up to 20 mg	Ca channel blocker	Potent negative inotropic effects and hypotension; avoid in HF

Notes:
- Vasopressin was removed from current guidelines to simplify given no advantage over epinephrine
- Adding methylprednisolone and vasopressin to epinephrine during ACLS plus stress dose hydrocortisone for post-ROSC shock may be considered to promote ROSC during cardiac arrest and improve discharge neurologic function in patients who survive; however further confirmatory data needed[5]
- When IV/IO access is unavailable, epinephrine, vasopressin, and lidocaine can be administered via endotracheal tube at 2–2.5 times the IV dose.

ACLS, Adult Advanced Cardiovascular life support; ADR, Adverse drug reaction; AF, Atrial fibrillation; AV, Atrioventricular note; Ca, Calcium; CPR, Cardiopulmonary resuscitation; DDI, Drug-drug interaction; EAD, Early afterdepolarization; ET, Endotracheal; HF, Heart failure; IO, Intraosseous; IV, Intravenous; K, Potassium; M, Myocardial infarction; MOA, Mechanism of action; Na, Sodium; NS, Normal saline; PEA, Pulseless electrical activity; pVT, Pulseless ventricular tachycardia; ROSC, Return of spontaneous circulation; VF, Ventricular fibrillation
Adapted from Panchal AR, Berg KM, Kudenchuk PJ, et al. 2018 American Heart Association focused update on advanced cardiovascular life support use of antiarrhythmic drugs during and immediately after cardiac arrest. Circulation. 2018;138:e740–e749 and Neumar RW, Otto CW, Link MS, et al. Part 8: adult advanced cardiovascular life support: 2010 American Heart Association Guidelines for Cardiopulmonary Resuscitation and Emergency Cardiovascular Care. Circulation. 2010;122(suppl 3):S729–S767.

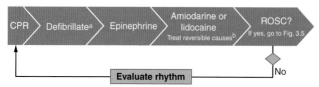

Figure 3.2 Algorithm for VF and pVT. *Data from Panchal AR, Berg KM, Kudenchuk PJ, et al. 2018 American Heart Association focused update on advanced cardiovascular life support use of antiarrhythmic drugs during and immediately after cardiac arrest. Circulation. 2018;138:e740–e749.* CPR, Cardiopulmonary resuscitation; *pVT,* Pulseless ventricular tachycardia; *ROSC,* Return of spontaneous circulation; *VF,* Ventricular fibrillation. [a]Biphasic, 120–200; escalate energy if initial dose <200. Monophasic: 360. [b]5 H's, **h**ypovolemia, **h**ypoxia, **h**ydrogen ion (acidosis), **h**ypo-/hyperkalemia, and **h**ypothermia. 5 T's, **t**ension pneumothorax, **t**amponade (cardiac), **t**oxins, **t**hrombosis (pulmonary), and **t**hrombosis (coronary).

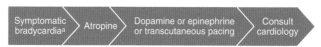

Figure 3.3 Algorithm for Bradycardia With Pulse. *Data from Neumar RW, Otto CW, Link MS, et al. Part 8: adult advanced cardiovascular life support: 2010 American Heart Association Guidelines for Cardiopulmonary Resuscitation and Emergency Cardiovascular Care. Circulation. 2010; 122(suppl 3):S729–S767.* [a]Symptoms: hypotension, altered mental status, shock, chest pain, or acute heart failure.

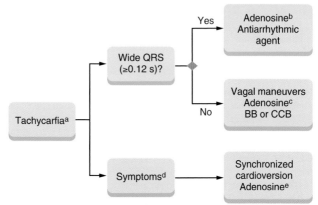

Figure 3.4 **Algorithm for Tachycardia with Pulse.** *Data from Neumar RW, Otto CW, Link MS, et al. Part 8: adult advanced cardiovascular life support: 2010 American Heart Association Guidelines for Cardiopulmonary Resuscitation and Emergency Cardiovascular Care. Circulation. 2010;122(suppl 3): S729–S767. BB,* β-blocker; *CCB,* Calcium channel blocker.
[a]Consider cardiology consultation.
[b]For regular and monomorphic tachycardia.
[c]For regular tachycardia.
[d]Hypotension, altered mental status, shock, chest pain, or acute heart failure.
[e]For regular narrow complex tachycardia.

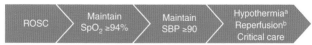

Figure 3.5 **Algorithm for Post-Cardiac Arrest Care.** *Data from Peberdy MA, Callaway CW, Neumar RW, et al. Part 9: post–cardiac arrest care: 2010 American Heart Association Guidelines for Cardiopulmonary Resuscitation and Emergency Cardiovascular Care. Circulation. 2010;122(suppl 3): S768–S786. AMI,* Acute myocardial infarction; *ROSC,* Return of spontaneous circulation; *SBP,* Systolic blood pressure; *SpO₂,* oxygen saturation; *STEMI,* ST-Elevation Myocardial Infarction. [a]Consider if patient comatose. [b]For STEMI/AMI.

Table 3.2 Common Vasoactive Infusions Used After Cardiac Arrest

DRUG	USUAL DOSE (mcg/kg/min)	CLINICAL PEARLS
Epinephrine	0.03–0.3	Mixed α and $\beta_{(1>2)}$ activity Used for SBP <90 mm Hg, symptomatic bradycardia, and hemodynamically unstable anaphylactic reactions Higher doses associated with increased α_1 activity
Norepinephrine	0.03–0.3	$\alpha > \beta_{(1>2)}$ activity; higher doses associated with increased α_1 activity Used for SBP <90 mm Hg Should be used in volume-resuscitated patients First line for septic shock
Phenylephrine	0.3–3	Pure α-agonist Used for SBP<90 mm Hg Should be used in volume-resuscitated patients Avoid in patients with low cardiac output
Dopamine	2–20	Dose-related receptor activity: 2–5 mcg/kg/min: dopamine receptor 5–10 mcg/kg/min: β_1-receptor >10 mcg/kg/min: α_1-receptor Can be arrhythmogenic at any dose Caution in patients with history of heart disease or arrhythmias Useful for patients with bradycardia and hypotension

Continued

Table 3.2 Common Vasoactive Infusions Used After Cardiac Arrest—cont'd

DRUG	USUAL DOSE (mcg/kg/min)	CLINICAL PEARLS
Dobutamine	2–20	Predominantly inotropic but with $\beta_1 > \beta_2 > \alpha_1$-receptor activity
		Used to treat low cardiac output
		α_1-agonist and β_2-agonist counterbalance→little change in SVR
		Can cause vasodilation in select patients
		Less systemic or pulmonary vasodilation than milrinone
		More tachycardia than milrinone but similar ventricular arrhythmias
		Caution in patients with history of arrhythmias
Milrinone	0.25–0.75	Phosphodiesterase type 3 inhibitor→increased intracellular cAMP→influx of calcium→inotropy and chronotropy
		Used to treat low cardiac output
		Loading dose rarely used because of hypotension
		Longer duration of activity compared to dobutamine
		Accumulation in renal dysfunction; renal adjustment needed
		More systemic and pulmonary vasodilation than dobutamine
		Less tachycardia than dobutamine but similar ventricular arrhythmias
		Caution in patients with history of arrhythmias

cAMP, Cyclic adenosine monophosphate; *SBP*, Systolic blood pressure; *SVR*, Systemic vascular resistance

Data from Peberdy MA, Callaway CW, Neumar RW, et al. Part 9: post–cardiac arrest care: 2010 American Heart Association guidelines for cardiopulmonary resuscitation and emergency cardiovascular care. *Circulation*. 2010;122(suppl 3):S768–S786.

Table 3.3 Complications of TTM and Management

COMPLICATIONS	MANAGEMENT
Shivering	Scheduled Acetaminophen 650 mg IV/NG/PR q4–6h or buspirone 30 mg NG q12h Magnesium sulfate 5 g IV over 5 h
Sedation and analgesia	Helps with shivering Adequate pain control and sedation recommended Target Richmond Agitation and Sedation Scale score -3 to -5 Accumulation during hypothermia: fentanyl, morphine, propofol, midazolam, rocuronium, vecuronium, and cisatracurium See Chapter 22 for details
Seizures	Same anticonvulsants for the treatment of status epilepticus caused by other etiologies may be considered after cardiac arrest Phenytoin: area under the concentration-time curve ↑ by 180% during hypothermia See Chapter 15 for details
Arrhythmias	Sinus bradycardia is common, thus should not be treated unless hypotension or organ dysfunction Caution in patients receiving medications that can prolong QT interval Consider discontinuing TTM if life-threatening arrhythmias
Hyperglycemia	Consider continuous insulin infusion to maintain blood glucose 140–180
Electrolyte abnormalities	Treat hypokalemia, hypomagnesemia, and hypophosphatemia Monitor electrolytes q3–4h Electrolyte shifts during cooling phase; reverse upon rewarming See Chapter 21 for details

IV, Intravenously; *NG*, Nasogastric; *PR*, Per rectum; *TTM*, Targeted temperature management
Data from Callaway CW, Donnino MW, Fink EL, et al. Part 8: post–cardiac arrest care: 2015 American Heart Association Guidelines Update for Cardiopulmonary Resuscitation and Emergency Cardiovascular Care. *Circulation.* 2015;132(suppl 2):S465–S482; and Neumar RW, Shuster M, Callaway CW, et al. Part 1: executive summary: 2015 American Heart Association Guidelines Update for Cardiopulmonary Resuscitation and Emergency Cardiovascular Care. *Circulation.* 2015;132(suppl 2):S315–S367.

References

1. Panchal AR, Berg KM, Kudenchuk PJ, et al. 2018 American Heart Association focused update on advanced cardiovascular life support use of antiarrhythmic drugs during and immediately after cardiac arrest. *Circulation*. 2018;138:e740–e749.

2. Neumar RW, Otto CW, Link MS, et al. Part 8: adult advanced cardiovascular life support: 2010 American Heart Association Guidelines for Cardiopulmonary Resuscitation and Emergency Cardiovascular Care. *Circulation*. 2010;122(suppl 3):S729–S767.

3. Peberdy MA, Callaway CW, Neumar RW, et al. Part 9: post–cardiac arrest care: 2010 American Heart Association Guidelines for Cardiopulmonary Resuscitation and Emergency Cardiovascular Care. *Circulation*. 2010;122(suppl 3):S768–S786.

4. Callaway CW, Donnino MW, Fink EL, et al. Part 8: post–cardiac arrest care: 2015 American Heart Association Guidelines Update for Cardiopulmonary Resuscitation and Emergency Cardiovascular Care. *Circulation*. 2015;132(suppl 2):S465–S482.

5. Neumar RW, Shuster M, Callaway CW, et al. Part 1: executive summary: 2015 American Heart Association Guidelines Update for Cardiopulmonary Resuscitation and Emergency Cardiovascular Care. *Circulation*. 2015;132(suppl 2):S315–S367.

4

Anticoagulation for Atrial Fibrillation or Atrial Flutter

This chapter will review the current recommendations from the American Heart Association/American College of Cardiology/Heart Rhythm Society practice guidelines.

ANTICOAGULATION TO PREVENT THROMBOEMBOLISM IN ATRIAL FIBRILLATION (AF) OR ATRIAL FLUTTER

Decisions Based on the Risk versus Benefit

- Risk of stroke (Table 4.1)
- Risk of bleeding (Table 4.2)

AF/Flutter ≥48 h or Unknown Duration

- Anticoagulate with warfarin (see Table 24.3) or non-vitamin K antagonist oral anticoagulant (NOAC) (Table 4.3) for at least 3 weeks before and 4 weeks after cardioversion.
- If urgent cardioversion required: anticoagulate as soon as possible and continue at least 4 weeks after cardioversion. Confirm absence of thrombus on the left side of the heart by transesophageal echocardiography before cardioversion.

Table 4.1 CHADS$_2$[a] and CHA$_2$DS$_2$-VASc[a] Stroke Risk Score in AF

RISK ASSESSMENT	SCORE	TOTAL PATIENT SCORE	ADJUSTED ANNUAL STROKE RATE (%)
CHADS$_2$			
Congestive heart failure	1	0	1.9
Hypertension	1	1	2.8
Age ≥75 yr	1	2	4.0
Diabetes mellitus	1	3	5.9
Stroke/TIA/thromboembolism	2	4	8.5
Maximum score	6	5	12.5
		6	18.2
CHA$_2$DS$_2$-VASc (Recommended)			
Congestive heart failure	1	0	0
Hypertension	1	1	1.3
Age ≥75 yr	2	2	2.2
Diabetes mellitus	1	3	3.2
Stroke/TIA/thromboembolism	2	4	4.0
Vascular disease	1	5	6.7
Age 65–74 yr	1	6	9.8
Sex category (female)	1	7	9.6
Maximum score	9	8	6.7
		9	15.2

Notes:
- CHA$_2$DS$_2$-VASc score of 0: no antithrombotic therapy reasonable
- CHA$_2$DS$_2$-VASc score of 1: no antithrombotic therapy or treatment with oral anticoagulant or aspirin reasonable
- Prior stroke, TIA, or CHA$_2$DS$_2$-VASc ≥2: anticoagulate with NOAC (preferred) or warfarin
- Warfarin is reasonable in chronic severe kidney disease or if contraindication to NOAC

AF, Atrial fibrillation; *NOAC*, Non-vitamin K antagonist oral anticoagulant; *TIA*, Transient ischemic attack
[a]Scoring not founded in the context of critically ill patients
From January CT, Wann LS, Alpert JS, et al. 2014 AHA/ACC/HRS guideline for the management of patients with atrial fibrillation: executive summary: a report of the American College of Cardiology/American Heart Association Task Force on Practice Guidelines and the Heart Rhythm Society. *Circulation.* 2014;130:2071–2104.

Table 4.2 HAS-BLED[a] or HEMORR$_2$ HAGES[a] Bleeding Risk
Scores in AF

RISK ASSESSMENT	SCORE	TOTAL PATIENT SCORE	BLEEDS/100 PATIENT-YEAR OF WARFARIN
HAS-BLED			
Hypertension	1	0	1.13
Abnormal renal/liver function	1 each	1	1.02
Stroke	1	2	1.88
Bleeding	1	3	3.74
Labile INRs while on warfarin	1	4	8.70
Elderly (age >65 yr)	1	5	12.5
Drugs (aspirin/NSAID) or alcohol	1 each	6	0
		Any score	1.56
HEMORR$_2$ HAGES			
Hepatic or renal disease	1	0	1.9
Ethanol abuse	1	1	2.5
Malignancy	1	2	5.3
Older age (>75 yr)	1	3	8.4
Reduced platelet count/function	1	4	10.4
Rebleeding risk	2	≥5	12.3
Hypertension (uncontrolled)	1	Any score	4.9
Anemia	1		
Genetic factors	1		
Excessive fall risk	1		
Stroke	1		

AF, Atrial fibrillation; *INRs*, International normalized ratios; *NSAIDS*, Nonsteroidal anti-inflammatory drugs.
[a]Scoring not founded in the context of critically ill patients
Adapted from Pisters R, Lane DA, Nieuwlaat R, et al. A novel user-friendly score (HAS-BLED) to assess 1-year risk of major bleeding in patients with atrial fibrillation: the Euro Heart Survey. *Chest*. 2010;138(5):1093–1100 and Gage BF, Yan Y, Milligan PE, et al. Clinical classification schemes for predicting hemorrhage: results from the National Registry of Atrial Fibrillation (NRAF). *Am Heart J*. 2006;151(3):713–719.

Table 4.3 Novel Oral Anticoagulants (NOAC) or Direct Oral Anticoagulants (DOAC)[a]

DRUG	STANDARD DOSING (PO)	RENAL DOSING (PO)	DRUG INTERACTION
Apixaban (Eliquis)	5 mg BID 2.5 mg BID if 2 of the following: Age ≥80 yr Weight ≤60 kg SCr ≥1.5 mg/dL	CrCl <25 or SCr >2.5: avoid use Not dialyzable	Avoid use with combined CYP3A4 and P-gp inducers (e.g., rifampin, phenytoin, carbamazepine, St. John's Wort) Combined strong CYP3A4 and P-gp inhibitors: reduce to 2.5 mg BID. If patient already on reduced dose, then avoid concurrent use
Dabigatran (Pradaxa)	150 mg BID	CrCl 30–50 and concomitant dronedarone or oral ketoconazole: 75 mg BID CrCl <30: avoid use	Avoid use with P-gp inducers (e.g., rifampin)
Edoxaban (Savaysa)	60 mg daily	CrCl >95: avoid use given reduced efficacy CrCl 15–50: 30 mg daily CrCl <15: avoid use Not dialyzable	Avoid use with combined CYP3A4 and P-gp inducers (e.g., rifampin, phenytoin, carbamazepine, St. John's Wort)

| **Rivaroxaban (Xarelto)** | 20 mg daily with evening meal; if concomitant clopidogrel, then 15 mg daily with food
Take with food to ↑ bioavailability | CrCl 15–50: 15 mg daily with evening meal
CrCl <15: avoid use | Avoid use with combined CYP3A4 and P-gp inducers (e.g., rifampin, phenytoin, carbamazepine, St. John's Wort)
Avoid use with combined strong CYP3A4 and P-gp inhibitors (e.g., ketoconazole, itraconazole, ritonavir) |

Notes:
- Concurrent aspirin or thienopyridine (e.g., clopidogrel, prasugrel, ticlopidine) increases bleeding
- Avoid prasugrel and ticagrelor
- Triple therapy (aspirin + thienopyridine + NOAC[a]) increases bleeding
- Anticoagulation reversal and antidotes (see Table 24.10)

BID, Two times daily; *CrCl*, Creatinine clearance using actual body weight; *CYP*, cytochrome P450 enzymes; *P-gp*, P-Glycoprotein; *PO*, Orally; *SCr*, Serum creatinine.
[a]DOAC and NOAC are used interchangeably

AF/Flutter <48 h

- High stroke risk: intravenous heparin (Table 4.4), low-molecular-weight heparin (Table 4.5), or NOAC (see Table 4.3) before or immediately after cardioversion, followed by long-term anticoagulation based on thromboembolic risk.
- Low stroke risk: no antithrombotic may be considered.

Table 4.4 Sample of Weight-Based IV Heparin Dosing Regimen

1. Give initial bolus 60 units/kg then continuous infusion 12 units/kg/h. Use adjusted body weight when patient is obese (≥20% above ideal body weight [IBW])

   Adjusted weight (kg) = IBW + 0.4 × (actual weight − IBW)

   Men: IBW (kg) = 50 + 2.3 × (height in inches >60 in)

   Women: IBW (kg) = 45 + 2.3 × (height in inches >60 in)

2. Check aPTT 6 h after start of infusion and adjust heparin dose as below:

aPTT (SECONDS)[a]	BOLUS DOSE	HOLD INFUSION	CONTINUOUS INFUSION
<35	60 units/kg	—	↑ by 4 units/kg/h
35–49	30 units/kg	—	↑ by 2 units/kg/h
50–84 (goal)	No change		
85–105	—	—	↓ by 2 units/kg/h
106–140	—	Hold for 1 h	↓ by 3 units/kg/h
>140	Hold and repeat aPTT q2h until aPTT <140		

[a]aPTT based on control value 29 s. aPTT goal and titration variable depending institution. Generally titrated to aPTT 1.5–2 times control.

3. Check aPTT 6 h after each dose adjustment. When aPTT at goal, monitor daily.

aPTT, Activated partial thromboplastin time; *IBW*, Ideal body weight; *IV*, Intravenous.

Table 4.5 Therapeutic LMWH (Off-Label Use)[a]

DRUG	STANDARD DOSING (SUBCUTANEOUS)	DOSE ADJUSTMENT
Dalteparin (Fragmin)	100–120 units/kg q12h Max 10,000 units per dose	Use with caution in severe renal impairment Not dialyzable
Enoxaparin (Lovenox)	1 mg/kg q12h	CrCl <30: 1 mg/kg q24h HD: avoid

CrCl, Creatinine clearance; *HD*, Hemodialysis; *LMWH*, Low-molecular-weight heparin
[a]Cardiac dosing based on mechanical heart valve to bridge anticoagulation and/or acute coronary syndromes

References

1. January CT, Wann LS, Alpert JS, et al. 2014 AHA/ACC/HRS guideline for the management of patients with atrial fibrillation: executive summary: a report of the American College of Cardiology/American Heart Association Task Force on Practice Guidelines and the Heart Rhythm Society. *Circulation*. 2014;130:2071–2104.

2. Pisters R, Lane DA, Nieuwlaat R, de Vos CB, Crijns HJ, Lip GY. A novel user-friendly score (HAS-BLED) to assess 1-year risk of major bleeding in patients with atrial fibrillation: the Euro Heart Survey. *Chest*. 2010;138(5):1093–1100.

3. Gage BF, Yan Y, Milligan PE, et al. Clinical classification schemes for predicting hemorrhage: results from the National Registry of Atrial Fibrillation (NRAF). *Am Heart J*. 2006;151(3):713–719.

5

Hypertensive Crisis

This chapter will review the pharmacotherapy for treatment of high blood pressure according to the 2017 High Blood Pressure Clinical Practice Guideline.

DEFINITIONS

Hypertensive Urgency

Severe elevations in blood pressure (>180/120 mm Hg) without target organ damage.

Hypertensive Emergency

Severe elevations in blood pressure (>180/120 mm Hg) with target organ dysfunction (e.g., chest pain, vision changes, acute kidney injury, aortic dissection, acute shortness of breath, heart failure exacerbation, obtundation).

MANAGEMENT

- Hypertensive crisis (Fig. 5.1)
- Hypertension in acute intracerebral hemorrhage (Fig. 5.2)
- Hypertension in acute ischemic stroke (Fig. 5.3)
- Drug therapy in hypertensive emergencies (Table 5.1)

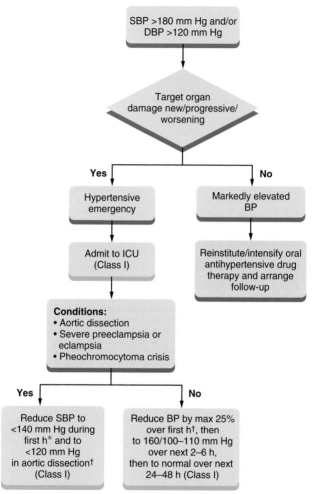

Figure 5.1 Diagnosis and Management of Hypertensive Crisis. *From Whelton PK, Carey RM, Aronow WS, et al. 2017 ACC/AHA/AAPA/ABC/ ACPM/AGS/APhA/ASH/ASPC/NMA/PCNA guideline for the prevention, detection, evaluation, and management of high blood pressure in adults: a report of the American College of Cardiology/American Heart Association Task Force on Clinical Practice Guidelines. J Am Coll Cardiol. 2018;71:e127– e248.* BP, blood pressure; *Class I*, Strong recommendation; *DBP*, Diastolic blood pressure; *ICU*, Intensive care unit; *SBP*, Systolic blood pressure. *Use medication specified in Table 5.1. †If other comorbidities present, select a medication specified in Table 5.1.

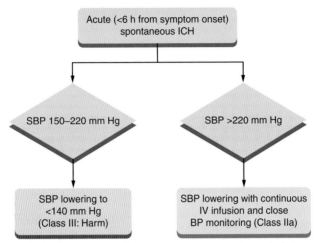

Figure 5.2 Management of Hypertension in Acute Intracerebral Hemorrhage (ICH). *From Whelton PK, Carey RM, Aronow WS, et al. 2017 ACC/ AHA/AAPA/ABC/ACPM/AGS/APhA/ASH/ASPC/NMA/PCNA guideline for the prevention, detection, evaluation, and management of high blood pressure in adults: a report of the American College of Cardiology/ American Heart Association Task Force on Clinical Practice Guidelines. J Am Coll Cardiol. 2018;71:e127–e248. BP,* Blood pressure; *Class IIa,* Can be beneficial; *Class III,* No benefit; *IV,* intravenous; *SBP,* systolic blood pressure.

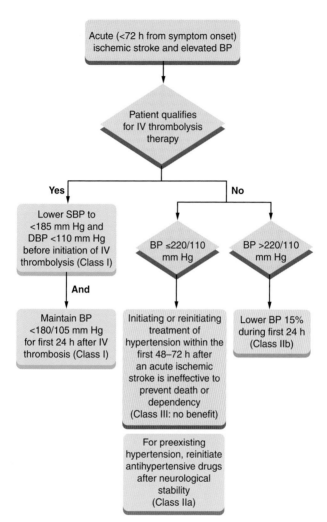

Figure 5.3 Management of Hypertension in Acute Ischemic Stroke. *From Whelton PK, Carey RM, Aronow WS, et al. 2017 ACC/AHA/AAPA/ABC/ ACPM/AGS/APhA/ASH/ASPC/NMA/PCNA guideline for the prevention, detection, evaluation, and management of high blood pressure in adults: a report of the American College of Cardiology/American Heart Association Task Force on Clinical Practice Guidelines. J Am Coll Cardiol. 2018;71:e127–e248. BP, Blood pressure; Class I, Strong recommendation; Class IIa, Moderate recommendation (can be beneficial); Class IIb, Weak recommendation; Class III, No benefit; DBP, Diastolic blood pressure; IV, intravenous; SBP, systolic blood pressure.*

Table 5.1 Classes of Drugs used for Treatment of Hypertensive Emergencies

DRUG	STANDARD DOSING (IV), PHARMACOKINETICS	SPECIAL INDICATIONS	COMMENTS
Vasodilators			
Nitroprusside (Nipride)	Start 0.3–0.5 mcg/kg/min, titrate by 0.5 mcg/kg/min q5min Max 10 mcg/kg/min Onset: seconds Duration: 1–2 min	Acute pulmonary edema	Liver failure: cyanide accumulation Renal failure: thiocyanate accumulation Toxicity associated with prolonged infusions (>72 h) or high doses (>3 mcg/kg/min) ADR: coronary steal, increased ICP Avoid in AMI, CAD, CVA, elevated ICP, renal/hepatic impairment
Nitroglycerin (Nitronal)	Start 5 mcg/min, titrate by 5 mcg/min q5min Max 100 mcg/min Onset: 2–5 min Duration: 5–10 min	Coronary ischemia/infarction Acute left ventricular failure Pulmonary edema Perioperative hypertension	Tachyphylaxis occurs rapidly Dose-limiting ADR: flushing, headache, erythema Veno > arterial vasodilator
Hydralazine	10–20 mg q4–6h prn Onset: 10 min Duration: 1–4 h	Eclampsia or preeclampsia	Prolonged and unpredictable hypotensive effect; second-line Risk of reflex tachycardia Headaches, lupus-like syndrome with chronic use

Dihydropyridine Calcium Channel Blockers

Nicardipine (Cardene)	Start 5 mg/h, titrate by 2.5 mg/h q5min Max 15 mg/h Onset: 5–10 min Duration: 2–4 h	Acute ischemic or hemorrhagic stroke Coronary ischemia/infarction Acute renal failure Eclampsia or preeclampsia Perioperative hypertension Catecholamine-induced hypertensive emergency (pheochromocytoma, interactions between MAOI and other drugs/food, clonidine withdrawal)	Risk of reflex tachycardia Infusion can lead to large fluid volume administered Caution: acute heart failure, coronary ischemia CI: aortic stenosis
Clevidipine (Cleviprex)	Start 1–2 mg/h, titrate by 1–2 mg/h q90s Max dose 32 mg/h Max duration 72 h Onset: 1–4 min Duration: 5–15 min	Acute ischemic or hemorrhagic stroke Acute pulmonary edema Acute renal failure Perioperative hypertension Catecholamine-induced hypertensive emergency	Formulated in oil-in-water formulation providing 2 kcal/mL of lipid calories Contains potential allergens (soy, egg)

Continued

Table 5.1 Classes of Drugs used for Treatment of Hypertensive Emergencies—cont'd

DRUG	STANDARD DOSING (IV), PHARMACOKINETICS	SPECIAL INDICATIONS	COMMENTS
β-Blockers			
Esmolol (Brevibloc)	Start 25 mcg/kg/min, titrate by 25 mcg/kg/min q5min Max 200 mcg/kg/min (bolus 500 mcg/kg rarely required given short onset) Onset: 1–2 min Duration: 10–20 min	Aortic dissection Coronary ischemia/infarction Perioperative hypertension	Ci: ADHF, reactive airways disease or COPD, heart block or bradycardia Use in conjunction with an arterial vasodilator for BP management in aortic dissection; initiate esmolol first due to delayed onset relative to vasodilators such as nitroprusside Useful in tachyarrhythmias Metabolized in blood by RBC esterases
Metoprolol	5–15 mg q5–15min prn Onset: 5–20 min Duration: 2–6 h	Aortic dissection Coronary ischemia/infarction	Ci: ADHF or bradycardia Use in conjunction with an arterial vasodilator for BP management in aortic dissection; initiate metoprolol first due to delayed onset relative to vasodilators such as nitroprusside Useful in tachyarrhythmias
Labetalol	20 mg, MR escalating doses 20–80 mg q10min prn, or 1 mg/min, titrate by 1 mg/min q2h Max 3 mg/min or total cumulative dose 300 mg Onset: 2–5 min Duration: 2–6 h	Acute ischemic or hemorrhagic stroke Aortic dissection Coronary ischemia/infarction Eclampsia or preeclampsia	Ci: ADHF, reactive airways disease or COPD, heart block or bradycardia May be used as monotherapy in acute aortic dissection Prolonged hypotension and/or bradycardia with overtreatment

α-Blocker			
Phentol- amine (OraVerse)	1–5 mg q5min prn Max 15 mg Onset: seconds Duration: 15 min	Catecholamine-induced hypertensive emergency	Use in catecholamine-induced hypertensive emergency
ACE Inhibitor			
Enalaprilat	1.25 mg q6h, titrate no more than q12–24h Max 5 mg q6h Onset: 15–30 min Duration: 6 h	Acute left ventricular failure	Avoid in AMI, bilateral renal artery stenosis, or pregnancy Caution in dose adjustments; slow onset and long duration of effect
Dopamine Agonist			
Fenoldopam (Corlopam)	0.1–0.3 mcg/kg/min, titrate by 0.05–0.1 mcg/kg/min q15min Max 1.6 mcg/kg/min Onset: 10–15 min Duration: 1 h	Most indications Preferred in acute renal failure	Risk of reflex tachycardia Caution: glaucoma or increased ICP Can cause hypokalemia, flushing

ACE, Angiotensin-converting enzyme; *ADHF*, Acute decompensated heart failure; *ADR*, Adverse drug reaction; *AMI*, Acute myocardial infarction; *BP*, Blood pressure; *CAD*, Coronary artery disease; *CI*, Contraindication; *COPD*, Chronic obstructive pulmonary disease; *CVA*, Cerebrovascular accident; *ICP*, Intracranial pressure; *IV*, Intravenously; *MAOI*, Monoamine oxidase inhibitors; *MR*, May repeat; *prn*, As needed; *RBC*, Red blood cell

Drugs without brand names are denoted by generic name only

Adapted from Whelton PK, Carey RM, Aronow WS, et al. 2017 ACC/AHA/AAPA/ABC/ACPM/AGS/APhA/ASH/ASPC/NMA/PCNA guideline for the prevention, detection, evaluation, and management of high blood pressure in adults: a report of the American College of Cardiology/American Heart Association Task Force on Clinical Practice Guidelines. *J Am Coll Cardiol.* 2018;71:e127–e248.

References

1. Whelton PK, Carey RM, Aronow WS, et al. 2017 ACC/AHA/AAPA/ABC/
    ACPM/AGS/APhA/ASH/ASPC/NMA/PCNA guideline for the prevention,
    detection, evaluation, and management of high blood pressure in adults:
    a report of the American College of Cardiology/American Heart
    Association Task Force on Clinical Practice Guidelines. *J Am Coll Cardiol.*
    2018;71:e127–e248.

Endocrine, Gastrointestinal, and Hepatic Disorders

6

Diabetic Ketoacidosis (DKA) and Hyperosmolar Hyperglycemic State (HHS)

This chapter will review the American Diabetes Association Practice Guidelines on diabetic ketoacidosis (DKA) and hyperosmolar hyperglycemic state (HHS).

INTRODUCTION

DKA and HHS are the two most serious acute complications of diabetes.

DIAGNOSIS CRITERIA (TABLE 6.1)

Table 6.1 Diagnostic Criteria for DKA and HHS

	NORMAL	DKA			HHS
		MILD	MODERATE	SEVERE	
Plasma glucose (mg/dL)	140–180	>250	>250	>250	>600
Arterial pH	7.38–7.44	7.25–7.30	7.00 to <7.24	<7.00	>7.30
Serum bicarbonate (mEq/L)	24–32	15–18	10 to <15	<10	>18
Urine ketones[a]	Negative	Positive	Positive	Positive	Small
Serum ketones	Negative	Positive	Positive	Positive	Small
Effective serum osmolality (mOsm/kg)	285–295	Variable	Variable	Variable	>320
Anion gap	<12	>10	>12	>12	Variable
Mental status	Alert	Alert	Alert/Drowsy	Stupor/Coma	Stupor/Coma

DKA, Diabetic ketoacidosis; *HHS*, Hyperosmolar hyperglycemic state
[a]A small amount can be present if fasting
Adapted from Kitabchi AE, Umpierrez GE, Miles JM, Fisher JN. Hyperglycemic crises in adult patients with diabetes. *Diabetes Care.* 2009;32(7):1335–1343 and Gosmanov AR, Gosmanova EO, Kitabchi AE. Hyperglycemic crises: diabetic ketoacidosis (DKA), and hyperglycemic hyperosmolar state (HHS). In: Feingold KR, Anawalt B, Boyce A, et al., eds. *Endotext* [Internet]. South Dartmouth, MA: MDText.com, Inc.; 2000. Available from: https://www.ncbi.nlm.nih.gov/books/NBK279052/. Updated May 17, 2018.

MANAGEMENT (TABLE 6.2)

Table 6.2 Goals and Management of DKA and HHS

I. Restore circulatory volume and tissue perfusion
   a. 0.9% NaCl at 1 L/h (15–20 mL/kg/h) during the first hour then 0.45% NaCl 250–500 mL/h (use 0.9% NaCl if corrected serum sodium <135)
   b. When blood glucose falls to 200 mg/dL (DKA) or 300 mg/dL (HHS), change to D5% 0.45% NaCl @ 150–250 mL/h
   c. Closely monitor and avoid fluid overload in renal or cardiac patients

II. Treat hyperglycemia
   a. IV insulin regular 0.1 unit/kg bolus then 0.1 unit/kg/h (DKA) or 0.05 unit/kg/h (HHS) (or 0.14 unit/kg/h without bolus)
   b. When blood glucose falls to 200 mg/dL (DKA) or 300 mg/dL (HHS), decrease insulin infusion to 0.02–0.05 unit/kg/h. Maintain blood glucose between 150 and 200 mg/dL until ketosis resolved (DKA) or between 200 and 300 mg/dL until patient is mentally alert (HHS)
   c. Transition to subcutaneous insulin after resolution of DKA or HHS. Overlap 1–2 h between subcutaneous and IV insulin.
   d. If hypoglycemia, glucose <70 mg/dL: D50% 50 mL IV q15min until glucose ≥70 mg/dL

III. Correct electrolyte abnormalities:
Potassium (K):
   a. If initial serum K < 3.3 mEq/L: hold insulin infusion and give K 20 mEq/h until K > 3.3 mEq/L
   b. If initial serum K 3.3–5.2: add 20–30 mEq K per liter of IV fluid to maintain K 4–5 mEq/L
   c. If initial serum K >5.2: do not give K but check serum K q2h
Bicarbonate:
   a. If pH <6.9 in DKA, give 100 mEq sodium bicarbonate in 400 mL sterile water over 2 h. If K ≤ 5.2, add 20 mEq K. Repeat q2h until pH ≥7
Phosphate:
   a. If serum phosphate < 1 mg/dL, 20–30 mEq/L sodium phosphate may be added to IV fluids. If K ≤ 5.2, K phosphate can replace sodium phosphate
   b. Maximal rate of phosphate replacement: 4.5 mmol/h

Continued

Table 6.2 Goals and Management of DKA and HHS—cont'd

IV. Treat underlying causes of DKA such as infection

Note on transitioning from IV to subcutaneous insulin:
- Patients previously on subcutaneous insulin: restart at previous dose and titrate as needed
- Insulin-naïve patients: consider a multidose insulin regimen at a dose 0.5–0.8 units/kg/day
  - Sample multidose regimen based on 70 kg at 0.5 units/kg/day:
    - NPH 12 units + regular 5 units BID before meals
    - Glargine or Detemir 20 units daily + Lispro, Aspart, or regular 5 units TID before meals

BID, Two times daily; *DKA*, Diabetic ketoacidosis; *HHS*, Hyperosmolar hyperglycemic state; *IV*, Intravenous; *K*, Potassium; *TID*, Three times daily

Adapted from References 1 and 2. Kitabchi AE, Umpierrez GE, Miles JM, Fisher JN. Hyperglycemic crises in adult patients with diabetes. *Diabetes Care*. 2009;32(7):1335–1343 and Gosmanov AR, Gosmanova EO, Kitabchi AE. Hyperglycemic crises: diabetic ketoacidosis (DKA), and hyperglycemic hyperosmolar state (HHS). In: Feingold KR, Anawalt B, Boyce A, et al., eds. *Endotext* [Internet]. South Dartmouth, MA: MDText.com, Inc.; 2000. Available from: https://www.ncbi.nlm.nih.gov/books/NBK279052/. Updated May 17, 2018.

INSULIN PREPARATIONS (TABLE 6.3)

Table 6.3 Pharmacokinetics of Insulin Preparations

INSULIN	PREPARATION	ONSET (h)	PEAK (h)	DURATION (h)
Rapid-acting	Aspart (Novolog)	<0.2	1–3	3–5
	Glulisine (Apidra)	0.3–0.4	1	4–5
	Lispro (Humalog)	0.25–0.5	0.5–2.5	≤5
Short-acting	Regular	0.5–1	2–3	3–6
Intermediate-acting	NPH	2–4	4–10	10–16
	Lente	3–4	4–12	12–18
Long-acting	Ultralente	6–10	10–16	18–20
	Detemir (Levemir)	2	3–9	6–24
	Glargine (Lantus)	2–4	Peakless	24
	Degludec (Tresiba)	2	Peakless	>40
Mixtures	Aspart protamine suspension + Aspart (Novolog mix 70/30)	0.25	1–4 (biphasic)	Up to 24
	Lispro protamine suspension + Lispro (Humalog Mix 75/25)	<0.25	1–3 (biphasic)	10–20
	NPH/Reg (Humulin 70/30, Humulin 50/50, Novolin 70/30)	0.5–1	2–10 (biphasic)	10–20

References

1. Kitabchi AE, Umpierrez GE, Miles JM, Fisher JN. Hyperglycemic crises in adult patients with diabetes. *Diabetes Care.* 2009;32(7):1335–1343.
2. Gosmanov AR, Gosmanova EO, Kitabchi AE. Hyperglycemic crises: diabetic ketoacidosis (DKA), and hyperglycemic hyperosmolar state (HHS). In: Feingold KR, Anawalt B, Boyce A, et al., eds. *Endotext.* South Dartmouth, MA: MDText.com, Inc.; 2000. Available from: https://www.ncbi.nlm.nih.gov/books/NBK279052/. Updated May 17, 2018.

7

Other Endocrine Emergencies

This chapter will review the pharmacologic management of adrenal and thyroid dysfunction according to the clinical practice guidelines and expert opinion.

THYROID STORM[1]

Definition

A life-threatening condition caused by an excess of thyroid hormone resulting in cardiovascular and central nervous system dysfunction and hyperpyrexia.

Precipitating Factors

- Abrupt discontinuation of antithyroid medications
- Acute illness (sepsis/infection, surgery or trauma)
- Graves' disease
- Radioiodine therapy
- Parturition
- Drugs (salicylates, amiodarone, anesthetics, pseudoephedrine)

Pharmacologic Management (Table 7.1)

Table 7.1 Pharmacologic Management of Thyroid Storm

DRUG	STANDARD DOSING	COMMENTS
Thionamides: Decrease Thyroid Hormone Synthesis		
Propylthiouracil	PO: 500–1000 mg ×1 then 250 mg q4h	First-line Decrease conversion of T4 to T3 Preferred in pregnant or lactating women ADR: agranulocytosis (rare), bleeding, hepatotoxicity, renal failure, vasculitis
Methimazole	PO: 20 mg q6–8h	For allergy or intolerance to propylthiouracil ADR: similar to propylthiouracil, but less hepatotoxicity than propylthiouracil
Iodine: Inhibit Thyroid Hormone Release		
Saturated solution of potassium iodide (SSKI)	PO: 5 drops q6h PR: 250–500 mg q6h	Start 1 h after thionamide started to prevent iodine serving as a substrate for new thyroid hormone production and worsening hyperthyroidism Use in conjunction with thionamides
Lugol solution	PO: 8 drops q6h PR: 5–10 drops q8–6h	
Lithium	PO: 300 mg q6–8h	Reserve for patients with iodine intolerance or CI Goal: 0.6–1 mEq/L Avoid in CrCl <30
β-Blockers: Control Heart Rate		
Propranolol	PO: 60–80 mg q4–6h IV: 0.5–1 mg over 10 min ×1 then 1–2 mg over 10 min PRN	Caution in congestive heart failure Decrease conversion of T4 to T3 at high doses Use with caution in renal/hepatic impairment

Table 7.1 Pharmacologic Management of Thyroid Storm—cont'd

DRUG	STANDARD DOSING	COMMENTS
Esmolol	250–500 mcg IV ×1 then 50–100 mcg/kg/min	Short-acting Rapid-titration
Bile Acid Sequestrants: Decrease Enterohepatic Recycling of Thyroid Hormones		
Cholestyramine	PO: 1–4 g BID	Off-label use. Use with a thionamide and propranolol
Glucocorticoids: Decrease Conversion of T4 to T3		
Hydrocortisone	IV: 300 mg ×1 then 100 mg q8h	Adjunct therapy Alternative: Dexamethasone 1–2 mg q6h

Note:
- Pyrexia: use acetaminophen instead of aspirin since aspirin can increase serum free T4 and T3

ADR, Adverse drug reaction; *BID*, Twice daily; *CI*, Contraindication; *CrCI*, Creatinine clearance; *IV*, Intravenously; *PO*, Orally; *PR*, Per rectum; *PRN*, As needed
Data from Ross DS, Burch HB, Cooper DS, et al. 2016 American Thyroid Association guidelines for diagnosis and management of hyperthyroidism and other causes of thyrotoxicosis. *Thyroid.* 2016;26(10):1343–1421.

MYXEDEMA COMA[2]

Definition

Severe hypothyroidism characterized by decreased mental status, hypothermia, cardiovascular instability, hyponatremia, hypoglycemia, and hypoventilation.

Risk Factors

- Noncompliance to thyroid replacement therapy
- Chronic hypothyroidism
- Infection
- Myocardial infarction
- Cold exposure
- Surgery
- Drugs (sedatives, opioids, amiodarone, lithium)

Management

- Supportive care
- Treat underlying etiology
- Pharmacologic management (Table 7.2)

Table 7.2 Pharmacologic Management of Myxedema Coma

DRUG	STANDARD DOSING (IV)	COMMENTS
Thyroid Hormone		
Levothyroxine T4	200–400 mcg ×1 then 50–100 mcg daily	Treat with both T4 and T3
		May discontinue T3 once patient stable
		Lower end of dosing range for smaller and older patients and coexisting cardiovascular disease
Liothyronine T3	5–20 mcg ×1 then 2.5–10 mcg q8h	Transition T4 to oral route as appropriate
		T4 bioavailability: 0.75
		Administer oral levothyroxine on empty stomach for optimal and consistent absorption
		Do not administer oral levothyroxine within 4h of calcium- or iron-containing products or bile acid sequestrants to avoid interaction
Glucocorticoids		
Hydrocortisone	100 mg q8h	Consider tapering dose after 2 days
		Discontinue if adrenal insufficiency ruled out

IV, Intravenously
Data from Jonklaas J, Bianco AC, Bauer AJ, et al. Guidelines for the treatment of hypothyroidism. *Thyroid.* 2014;24(12):1670–1751.

ADRENAL CRISIS[3]

Definition

Acute adrenal insufficiency, most common in patients with primary adrenal insufficiency, characterized by severe weakness, syncope, psychosis, or altered mental status mimicking sepsis.

Predisposing Factors

- Previously undiagnosed primary adrenal insufficiency precipitated by infection or stress
- Glucocorticoid therapy noncompliance during infection or major illness or persistent vomiting
- Bilateral adrenal infarction or hemorrhage
- Acute cortisol deficiency due to pituitary apoplexy or abrupt discontinuation of chronic steroid therapy
- Drugs that inhibit cortisol synthesis: etomidate, ketoconazole
- Drugs that accelerate cortisol metabolism: phenytoin, rifampin

Management

- 0.9% NaCl or D5% 0.9% NaCl 2–3 L within 12–24 h based on volume status
- Hydrocortisone (Solu-Cortef) 100 mg IV ×1 then 200 mg/day (continuous IV infusion or q6h injection). If hydrocortisone unavailable, use prednisolone. Dexamethasone least preferred because of risk of cushingoid side effects due to difficult dose titration.
- Comparison of systemic corticosteroids (Table 7.3)
- Fludrocortisone 0.1 mg PO daily after 0.9% NaCl completed
- Stress-dose steroids to prevent adrenal crisis in patients on chronic steroid use (Table 7.4)
- After initial treatment and patient stabilized, adrenocorticotropic hormone (ACTH) stimulation test can be performed to confirm diagnosis of primary adrenal insufficiency (Box 7.1)

Table 7.3 Comparison of Systemic Corticosteroids

CORTICOSTEROIDS	EQUIVALENT DOSES (mg)	RELATIVE POTENCY: ANTI-INFLAMMA-TORY	RELATIVE POTENCY: MINER-ALOCORTI-COID	DURA-TION OF ACTION (h)
Hydrocortisone	20	1	2	8–12
Cortisone acetate	25	0.8	2	"
Prednisone	5	4	1	12–36
Prednisolone	5	4	1	"
Methylprednisolone	4	5	0	"
Triamcinolone	4	5	0	"
Dexamethasone	0.75	20–30	0	36–72
Betamethasone	0.6–0.75	20–30	0	"
Fludrocortisone	—	10	125	12–36

Notes:
- In septic shock, hydrocortisone can be tapered off over a few days after vasopressor therapy is no longer required and serum lactate levels are normalized
- Generally, intravenous glucocorticoid therapy can be tapered over 1–3 days and transitioned to oral stress or maintenance dose
- Physiologic hydrocortisone range: 10–20 mg in AM and 5–10 mg in PM
- Fludrocortisone supplementation not needed unless aldosterone deficiency
- For primary adrenal insufficiency or potassium >6 mEq/L: hydrocortisone is preferred over dexamethasone due to its mineralocorticoid property.

From Brunton LL, Chabner BA, Knollmann BC, eds. In: Brunton LL, Chabner BA, Knollmann BC, eds. *Goodman & Gilman's: The Pharmacological Basis of Therapeutics.* 12th ed. McGraw-Hill Education; 2011 (Chapter 42).

Table 7.4 Stress-Dose Steroids to Prevent Adrenal Crisis in Patients on Chronic Steroids

TYPE OF PROCEDURE/STRESS	HYDROCORTISONE (OR EQUIVALENT) ON DAY OF PROCEDURE
Minor (colonoscopy, gastroenteritis, laparoscopic procedure)	25 mg
Moderate (severe gastroenteritis, pneumonia, febrile illness, open abdominal surgeries)	50–75 mg
Severe (cardiovascular surgery, Whipple procedure, pancreatitis, active labor)	100–150 mg

Note:
Taper to usual dose over 1–2 days if clinically appropriate

Data from Bornstein SR, Allolio B, Arlt W, et al. Diagnosis and treatment of primary adrenal insufficiency: an endocrine society clinical practice guideline. *J Clin Endocrinol Metab.* 2016;101:364–389.

Box 7.1 ACTH Stimulation Test

BASELINE PLASMA CORTISOL LEVEL	COMMENTS
<5 µg/dL	Adrenal insufficiency
≥ 5 µg/dL	Perform ACTH stimulation test: Cosyntropin 250 mcg IV ×1 then check peak cortisol level 0.5–1 h after • Plasma cortisol <18 µg/dL: adrenal insufficiency • Plasma cortisol ≥ 18 µg/dL: normal response, however does not eliminate adrenal suppression

ACTH, Adrenocorticotropic hormone; *IV,* Intravenously
Data from Bornstein SR, Allolio B, Arlt W, et al. Diagnosis and treatment of primary adrenal insufficiency: an Endocrine Society clinical practice guideline. *J Clin Endocrinol Metab.* 2016;101:364–389.

References

1. Ross DS, Burch HB, Cooper DS, et al. 2016 American Thyroid Association guidelines for diagnosis and management of hyperthyroidism and other causes of thyrotoxicosis. *Thyroid.* 2016;26(10):1343–1421.
2. Jonklaas J, Bianco AC, Bauer AJ, et al. Guidelines for the treatment of hypothyroidism. *Thyroid.* 2014;24(12):1670–1751.
3. Bornstein SR, Allolio B, Arlt W, et al. Diagnosis and treatment of primary adrenal insufficiency: an Endocrine Society clinical practice guideline. *J Clin Endocrinol Metab.* 2016;101:364–389.
4. Brunton LL, Chabner BA, Knollmann BC, eds. *Goodman & Gilman's: The Pharmacological Basis of Therapeutics.* 12th ed. McGraw-Hill Education; New York, NY, 2011 (Chapter 42).

8

Gastroenterology

This chapter will review the pharmacotherapy for management of gastrointestinal (GI) fistulas, postoperative ileus, nausea, and vomiting and upper GI bleeding according to expert opinion.

GI FISTULAS[1]

Definition

An abnormal connection between the GI track and the skin, another internal organ, or an internal cavity.

Causes

- Postoperative fistulas (most common; 80%)
- Spontaneous fistulas (Crohn disease and inflammatory bowel disease are the leading cause)
- Trauma-induced fistulas

Management

- Fluid resuscitation and electrolyte management (see Chapter 21)
- Drainage
- Nutrition (enteral vs. parenteral)
- Octreotide
  - Mimics natural somatostatin found in the GI by inhibiting hormone secretion, exocrine secretory response,

GI motor activity, and nutrient absorption and stimulation of water and electrolyte absorption.

- Dose: 100 mcg subcutaneously three times daily
- Discontinue if no response within 48 h

POSTOPERATIVE ILEUS (POI)[2]

Definition

A transient GI dysmotility following a surgery.

Causes

- Increased sympathetic stimulation postoperatively
- Damage to the vagal nerve during abdominal surgery
- Inflammation of the GI tract after surgery
- Drugs: anesthetics, opioids, anticholinergics

Pharmacologic Management (Table 8.1)

Table 8.1 Pharmacologic Management of POI

DRUG	STANDARD DOSING	COMMENTS
Opioid-Sparing Analgesic Agents: NSAIDs		
Ketorolac (Toradol) 15 mg, 30 mg injection	15–30 mg IV q6h PRN Max: 5 days	Opioid sparing via analgesic and anti-inflammatory effects. Need to ensure adequate hydration prior to NSAID use. CrCl <30: avoid use
Ibuprofen (Caldolor) 800 mg injection	400–800 mg IV q6h PRN	
Diclofenac (Dyloject) 37.5 mg injection	37.5 mg IV q6h PRN	"
Laxatives		
Bisacodyl (Dulcolax) 10 mg suppository	10 mg rectally daily	Stimulant laxative

Table 8.1 Pharmacologic Management of POI—cont'd

DRUG	STANDARD DOSING	COMMENTS
Peripherally Acting Mu-Opioid Receptor Antagonists		
Alvimopan (Entereg) 12 mg capsule	12 mg PO 0.5–5 h prior to surgery, followed by 12 mg BID beginning the day after surgery up to 7 days	FDA approved for POI 200-fold selectivity for the peripheral opioid receptors Poor GI/systemic absorption REMS drug
Methylnaltrexone (Relistor) 8 mg, 12 mg injection	0.15 mg/kg SubQ daily or every other day	FDA approved for chronic opioid-induced consti-pation, not POI. Does not affect opioid anal-gesic effects. Does not cross the blood-brain barrier. Discontinue all laxatives prior to use; restart laxatives PRN if suboptimal response to methylnaltrexone or naloxegol after 3 days
Naloxegol (Movantik) 12.5 mg, 25 mg tablet	25 mg PO daily 12.5 mg if 25 mg not tolerated	
Prokinetic Agents		
Erythromycin (Erythrocin) 250 mg, 500 mg tablet 500 mg injection 200–400 mg/5 mL oral suspension	IV: 3 mg/kg over 45 min q8h PO: 250–500 mg (base) TID AC	Macrolide antibiotic with prokinetic activity Off-label use; inconsistent data Erythromycin ethylsuc-cinate 400 mg = erythromycin base or stearate 250 mg
Metoclopramide (Reglan) 10 mg injection 5 mg, 10 mg tablet 1 mg/mL oral solution	PO, IM, IV, SubQ: 5–10 mg BID–TID AC PO route preferred	Prokinetic and antiemetic activity Off-label use; inconsistent data Decrease dose by 50% in CrCl <40 (IV) and CrCl ≤60 (PO)

Continued

Table 8.1 Pharmacologic Management of POI—cont'd

DRUG	STANDARD DOSING	COMMENTS
Prucalopride (Motegrity) 1 mg, 2 mg tablet	2 mg PO daily CrCl <30: 1 mg PO daily ESRD on HD: avoid	Serotonin 5-HT4 receptor agonist Off-label use Start before surgery ADR: headache, abdominal pain, nausea, diarrhea
Tegaserod (Zelnorm) 2 mg, 6 mg tablet	Females <65 years: 6 mg PO BID AC (dosing for IBSC or CIC)	Serotonin 5-HT4 receptor agonist FDA approved for emergency treatment of IBSC and CIC in women <55 years without alternative therapy option

AC, Before meals; *ADR*, Adverse drug reaction; *BID*, Twice daily; *CIC*, Chronic idiopathic constipation; *CrCl*, Creatinine clearance; *ESRD*, End stage renal disease; *5-HT4*, 5-Hydroxytryptamine receptor 4; *FDA*, Food and Drug Administration; *GI*, Gastrointestinal; *HD*, Hemodialysis; *IBSC*, Irritable bowel syndrome with constipation; *IM*, Intramuscular; *IV*, Intravenous; *NSAID*, Nonsteroidal anti-inflammatory drug; *PO*, Orally; *POI*, Postoperative ileus; *PRN*, As needed; *REMS*, Risk evaluation and mitigation strategies; *SubQ*, Subcutaneously; *TID*, Three times daily
Data from Schwenk ES, Grant AE, Torjman MC, et al. The efficacy of peripheral opioid antagonists in opioid-induced constipation and postoperative ileus: a systematic review of the literature. *Reg Anesth Pain Med.* 2017;42:767–777.

POSTOPERATIVE NAUSEA AND VOMITING (PONV)[3]

Definition

Nausea, vomiting, or retching in the immediate 24 postoperative hours.

Risk of PONV (Table 8.2)

Table 8.2 Risk of PONV

Risk factors	Female gender
	Nonsmoker
	History of motion sickness or previous PONV
	Expected administration of postoperative opioids
No risk factor (low risk)	10% of PONV
One risk factor (low risk)	20% of PONV
Two risk factors (medium risk)	40% of PONV
Three risk factors (medium risk)	60% of PONV
Four risk factors (high risk)	80% of PONV

PONV, Postoperative nausea and vomiting
Data from Apfel CC, Koivuranta EM, Greim CA, et al. A simplified risk score for predicting postoperative nausea and vomiting: conclusions from cross-validations between two centers. *Anesthesiology*. 1999;91(3):693–700.

Management of PONV

- Treatment algorithm according to risk factors (Fig. 8.1)
- Pharmacologic management (Table 8.3)

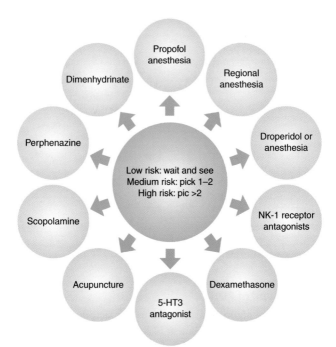

Figure 8.1 Treatment Algorithm for Postoperative Nausea and Vomiting According to Risk Factors. *NK-1*, Neurokinin-1; *5-HT3*, 5-Hydroxytryptamine receptor 3. *Data from Gan TJ, Diemunsch P, Habib AS. Consensus guidelines for the management of postoperative nausea and vomiting. Anesth Analg. 2014;118:85–113.*

Table 8.3 Pharmacologic Prophylaxis of Postoperative Nausea and Vomiting

DRUG	STANDARD DOSING	TIMING	COMMENTS
Serotonin-3 Antagonists (5-HT3 Antagonist): First-Line			
Ondansetron (Zofran) 4 mg, 8 mg ODT and oral film 4 mg injection	4 mg IV 8 mg PO 30–60 min before surgery[a]	End of surgery	All except for palonosetron can cause QT prolongation. Palonosetron has a longer half-life of 40 h compared to others. Can be combined with droperidol or dexamethasone for moderate-high risk for PONV
Granisetron (Sustol) 0.1 mg, 1 mg, 4 mg injection	0.35–3 mg IV	End of surgery	
Palonosetron (Aloxi) 0.25 mg injection	0.075 mg IV	Start of surgery	
Corticosteroids			
Dexa-methasone (Decadron) 10 mg injection	4–8 mg IV	Start of surgery	Caution in diabetes due to risk of hyperglycemia. Efficacy of dexamethasone 4 mg IV similar to ondansetron 4 mg IV and droperidol 1.25 mg IV. Combine droperidol with dexamethasone for high risk of PONV.
Methylpred-nisolone (Solume-drol) 40 mg, 80 mg, 125 mg injection	40 mg IV	—	

Continued

Table 8.3 Pharmacologic Prophylaxis of Postoperative Nausea and Vomiting—cont'd

DRUG	STANDARD DOSING	TIMING	COMMENTS
Neurokinin Receptor Antagonist (NK-1 Receptor Antagonist)			
Aprepitant (Emend) 40, 80, 125 mg capsule 125 mg oral suspension	40–80 mg PO	Start of surgery	Half-life of 40 h
Rolapitant (Varubi) 90 mg	90 mg PO	Start of surgery	Half-life of 180 h FDA approved for chemotherapy-induced N/V only
Butyrophenones: Second-Line			
Droperidol (generic) 2.5 mg injection	0.625–1.25 mg IV	End of surgery	Risk of QTc prolongation; monitor ECG. Efficacy of droperidol 1.25 mg IV similar to ondansetron 4 mg IV and dexamethasone 4 mg IV. Combine droperidol with dexamethasone for high risk of PONV
Haloperidol (Haldol) 5 mg injection	0.5–2 mg IM/IV IV: off-label use	Start or end of surgery	
Antihistamines			
Dimenhydrinate (Dramamine) 50 mg injection	1 mg/kg IV	—	Lack of data

Table 8.3 Pharmacologic Prophylaxis of Postoperative Nausea and Vomiting—cont'd

DRUG	STANDARD DOSING	TIMING	COMMENTS
Meclizine (Bonine) 12.5 mg, 25 mg	50 mg PO	—	Combine with ondansetron 4 mg IV
Anticholinergic Agent: Adjunct			
Scopolamine patch (Transderm Scop) 1.5 mg patch 72 h	Apply one patch behind the ear; remove 24 h after surgery	Prior evening or 2–4 h before surgery	ADR: visual disturbances, dry mouth, dizziness Scopolamine combined with ondansetron or dexamethasone more effective than scopolamine alone
Phenothiazines			
Perphenazine (generic) 2 mg, 4 mg, 8 mg, 16 mg	2.5–5 mg IV/IM	—	Injection not available in U.S.
Metoclo-pramide (Reglan) 10 mg injection	25–50 mg IV	30–60 min before surgery	Risk of dyskinesia or EPS
Prochlor-perazine (Compro) 10 mg injection	5–10 mg IV	End of surgery	Most effective for opioid-induced N/V ADR: sedation and EPS

Continued

Table 8.3 Pharmacologic Prophylaxis of Postoperative Nausea and Vomiting—cont'd

DRUG	STANDARD DOSING	TIMING	COMMENTS

Notes:
- Rescue therapy within the first 6 h postoperatively: recommend an antiemetic from different class from the initial prophylactic drug
- Rescue therapy after the first 6 h postoperatively: repeat doses of the initial drug may be used (do not readminister dexamethasone, aprepitant, palonosetron or scopolamine)
- If no prophylactic agent given: recommend a serotonin-3 antagonist at a lower dose
- Propofol: a sedative-hypnotic used for induction and maintenance of general anesthesia has antiemetic properties
- Midazolam 2 mg IV 30 min before end of surgery may be as effective as ondansetron 4 mg IV

ADR, Adverse drug reaction; *ECG*, Electrocardiogram; *EPS*, Extrapyramidal symptoms; *FDA*, Food and Drug Administration; *IM*, Intramuscular; *IV*, Intravenous; *N/V*, Nausea/vomiting; *ODT*, Oral disintegrating tablet; *PO*, orally; *PONV*, postoperative nausea and vomiting
ᵃUse oral disintegrating tablet or oral soluble film
From Schwenk ES, Grant AE, Torjman MC, et al. The efficacy of peripheral opioid antagonists in opioid-induced constipation and postoperative ileus: a systematic review of the literature. *Reg Anesth Pain Med.* 2017;42:767–777.

UPPER GI BLEEDING (UGIB)[5-7]
Definition
Bleeding within the GI track proximal to the jejunum.

Causes
- Nonvariceal hemorrhage (e.g., gastric/duodenal ulcer, gastroduodenal erosions, Mallory-Weiss tear)
- Variceal hemorrhage (gastroesophageal varices present in ~50% of patients with cirrhosis)

Pharmacologic Management
Nonvariceal UGIB
- Gastric acid inhibits platelet aggregation and promotes fibrinolysis; therefore, gastric acid-suppression with proton pump inhibitors to raise intragastric pH acid recommended

- Esomeprazole or pantoprazole 80 mg intravenous (IV) bolus, followed by 8 mg/h ×72 h or 40 mg IV q12h with/without loading dose of 80 mg

Variceal UGIB

- Octreotide induces splanchnic vasoconstriction thereby decreasing variceal blood flow and hemorrhage
- Octreotide 50 mcg IV bolus, followed by 50 mcg/h ×3–5 days
- Esomeprazole or pantoprazole 80 mg IV bolus, followed by 8 mg/h until variceal UGIB is confirmed

Cirrhosis ± ascites and UGIB

- Ceftriaxone 1 g IV daily (up to 7 days) until hemorrhage resolved and octreotide discontinued

Nonselective β-blocker (propranolol, nadolol, carvedilol)

- Consider after octreotide discontinued

Bleeding due to anticoagulation: see Table 24.10 for reversal agents

H. pylori treatment (Table 8.4)

Table 8.4 Initial Antibiotic Therapy for *Helicobacter Pylori* Infection

REGIMEN/DOSE	DOSING FREQUENCY	DURATION (DAYS)	COMMENTS
Bismuth Quadruple Therapy			
Bismuth 300 mg	QID	10–14	For prior exposure to macrolides, local clarithromycin resistance, or penicillin allergy
Metronidazole 250–500 mg	QID		
Tetracycline 500 mg[a]	QID		
PPI (standard dose) (Pylera: bismuth + metronidazole + tetracycline combination)	BID		

Continued

Table 8.4 Initial Antibiotic Therapy for *Helicobacter Pylori* Infection—cont'd

REGIMEN/DOSE	DOSING FREQUENCY	DURATION (DAYS)	COMMENTS
Clarithromycin Triple Therapy			
Clarithromycin 500 mg	BID	14	—
Amoxicillin 1 g	BID		
PPI	BID		
Clarithromycin 500 mg	BID	14	For penicillin allergy
Metronidazole 500 mg	TID		
PPI (standard/double dose)	BID		
Concomitant Therapy			
Clarithromycin 500 mg	BID	10–14	—
Amoxicillin 1 g	BID		
Nitroimidazole[b] 500 mg	BID		
PPI (standard dose)	BID		
Sequential Therapy			
Amoxicillin 1 g + PPI (standard dose) then	BID	5–7	Complex regimen
Clarithromycin 500 mg + Nitroimidazole[b] 500 mg + PPI	BID	5–7	"
Hybrid Therapy			
Amoxicillin 1 g + PPI (standard dose) then	BID	7	Complex regimen
Amoxicillin + clarithromycin 500 mg + nitroimidazole[b] 500 mg + PPI	BID	7	"

Table 8.4 Initial Antibiotic Therapy for *Helicobacter Pylori* Infection—cont'd

REGIMEN/DOSE	DOSING FREQUENCY	DURATION (DAYS)	COMMENTS
Levofloxacin Triple Therapy			
Levofloxacin 500 mg	Daily	10–14	Metronidazole: substitute for amoxicillin in penicillin allergy
Amoxicillin 1 g	BID		
PPI (standard dose)	BID		
Levofloxacin Sequential Therapy			
Amoxicillin 1 g + PPI (standard/double dose), then	BID	5–7	Complex regimen
Levofloxacin 500 mg QD + nitroimidazole[b] 500 mg + amoxicillin + PPI	BID	5–7	"
LOAD[c]			
Levofloxacin 250 mg	Daily	7–10	Limited data
Nitazoxanide 500 mg	BID		
Doxycycline 100 mg	Daily		
PPI (double dose)	Daily		
PPI Standard Dosing			
Esomeprazole 20 mg	BID		
Lansoprazole 30 mg	BID		
Omeprazole 20 mg	BID		
Pantoprazole 40 mg	BID		

BID, Twice daily; *PPI*, Proton pump inhibitor; *QD*, Daily; *QID*, Four times daily; *TID*, Three times daily
[a]Doxycyclin 100 mg BID may be substituted if tetracycline unavailable
[b]Metronidazole or tinidazole
[c]Levofloxacin, omeprazole, nitazoxanide (Alinia), doxycycline
From Chey WD, Leontiadis GI, Howden CW, Moss SF. ACG clinical guideline: treatment of *Helicobacter pylori* infection. *Am J Gastroenterol.* 2017;112:212–238.

References

1. Coughlin S, Roth L, Lurati G, Faulhaber M. Somatostatin analogues for the treatment of enterocutaneous fistulas: a systematic review and meta-analysis. *World J Surg.* 2012;36:1016–1029.
2. Schwenk ES, Grant AE, Torjman MC, McNulty SE, Baratta JL, Viscusi ER. The efficacy of peripheral opioid antagonists in opioid-induced constipation and postoperative ileus: a systematic review of the literature. *Reg Anesth Pain Med.* 2017;42:767–777.
3. Gan TJ, Diemunsch P, Habib AS, et al. Consensus guidelines for the management of postoperative nausea and vomiting. *Anesth Analg.* 2014;118:85–113.
4. Apfel CC, Koivuranta EM, Greim CA, Roewer N. A simplified risk score for predicting postoperative nausea and vomiting: conclusions from cross-validations between two centers. *Anesthesiology.* 1999;91(3):693–700.
5. Hwang JH, Shergill AK, Acosta RD, et al.; American Society for Gastrointestinal Endoscopy. The role of endoscopy in the management of variceal hemorrhage. *Gastrointest Endosc.* 2014;80(2):221–227.
6. Hwang JH, Fisher DA, Ben-Menachem T, et al.; Standards of Practice Committee of the American Society for Gastrointestinal Endoscopy. The role of endoscopy in the management of acute non-variceal upper GI bleeding. *Gastrointest Endosc.* 2012;75(6):1132–1138.
7. Laine L, Jensen DM. Management of patients with ulcer bleeding. *Am J Gastroenterol.* 2012;107:345–360.
8. Chey WD, Leontiadis GI, Howden CW, Moss SF. ACG clinical guideline: treatment of *Helicobacter pylori* infection. *Am J Gastroenterol.* 2017;112: 212–238.

9

Severe Acute Pancreatitis and Liver Failure

This chapter will review the pharmacotherapy for management of severe acute pancreatitis and liver failure according to the American College of Gastroenterology and American Association for the Study of Liver Diseases guidelines.

SEVERE ACUTE PANCREATITIS[1]

Definition

Pancreatitis associated with hypovolemia, organ failure, or local complications including necrosis, abscess, or pseudocyst.

Management

- Fluid resuscitation
  - Isotonic crystalloid 250–500 mL/h
  - Caution in cardiovascular and/or renal disease
  - Aggressive intravenous hydration most beneficial first 12–24 h
- Pain control
  - Intravenous (IV) hydromorphone 0.1–0.4 mg q10min as needed (PRN)
  - IV fentanyl 20–50 mcg q10min PRN
- Endoscopic retrograde cholangiopancreatography (ERCP)
  - Indicated in selected acute pancreatitis with concomitant acute cholangitis

- Postprocedure rectal nonsteroidal anti-inflammatory (NSAID) suppositories: indomethacin 100 mg ×1 immediately after ERCP
- Antibiotics
  - Indicated in extrapancreatic infection (e.g., cholangitis, bloodstream infections, pneumonia, urinary tract infections) and infected necrosis
  - Empiric antibiotic therapy for extrapancreatic infection: see Chapter 11
  - Empiric antibiotic therapy for infected necrosis (Table 9.1)
- Nutrition support
  - Enteral feeding recommended
  - Parenteral nutrition only if enteral feeding not tolerated or inadequate
- Surgery
  - Urgent or delayed surgical intervention based on expert opinion

LIVER FAILURE[2]

Definitions

- Acute liver failure (ALF) is defined as evidence of coagulopathy (e.g., International normalized ratio ≥1.5) and mental status change in a patient without preexisting liver failure and with an illness duration <26 weeks. ALF is a rare condition with an annual incidence of <10 cases per million population in the developed world.
- Acute-on-chronic liver failure: most cases of liver failure involve patients with chronic liver disease (cirrhosis) who develop an acute deterioration of liver function and organ failure usually precipitated by an infection. Management below focuses on this group of patients.

Pharmacologic Management

Spontaneous bacterial peritonitis (SBP)

- Infection in the ascitic fluid
  - Pathogens: 75% gram-negative aerobic bacilli (*Escherichia coli* and *Klebsiella pneumoniae*) and 25% gram-positive aerobic cocci (*Streptococcus pneumoniae*)

Table 9.1 Empiric Antibiotic Therapy for Infected Necrosis

ANTIBIOTICS	STANDARD DOSING (IV)	RENAL DOSING	COMMENTS
Carbapenems			
Doripenem (Doribax) 250 mg, 500 mg	500 mg q8h	CrCl 30–50: 250 mg q8h CrCl 11–29: 250 mg q12h HD: 250 mg q24h[a]; if PSA, 500 mg q12h ×1 day then 500 mg q24h[a]	Similar spectrum of activity as meropenem except more potent in vitro activity against PSA than meropenem
Ertapenem (Invanz) 1 g	1 g q24h	CrCl ≤30 and HD: 500 mg daily	Compared to imipenem/meropenem, less active against PSA, *acinetobacter, enterococci,* and Pcn-resistant *pneumococci*
Imipenem-cilastatin (Primaxin) 250 mg, 500 mg	500 mg to 1 g q6h	CrCl 60–89: 500–750 mg q8h CrCl 30–59: 500 mg q6–8h CrCl 15–29 and HD: 500 mg q12h[a] CrCl <15 without HD: avoid use	Imipenem: consider decreasing dose in patients <70 kg to prevent seizures
Meropenem (Merrem) 500 mg, 1 g	1 g q8h	CrCl 26–50: same dose q12h CrCl 10–25: half dose q12h CrCl <10: half dose q24h HD: 500 mg q24h[a]	Similar spectrum of activity as imipenem; slightly lower risk of seizures than imipenem

Continued

Table 9.1 Empiric Antibiotic Therapy for Infected Necrosis—cont'd

ANTIBIOTICS	STANDARD DOSING (IV)	RENAL DOSING	COMMENTS
Antipseudomonal Cephalosporins			
Cefepime (Maxipime) 1 g, 2 g	2 g q8–12h	CrCl 30–60: 2 g q12–24h CrCl <30: 1–2 g q24h HD: 0.5–1 g q24h[a]	Must be combined with metronidazole for anaerobic coverage 10% cross sensitivity with Pcn allergy
Ceftazidime (Fortaz) 500 mg, 1 g, 2 g	2 g q8h	CrCl 31–50: 2 g q12h CrCl 16–30: 2 g q24h CrCl ≤15 & HD: 1 g q24h[a]	
Fluoroquinolones			
Ciprofloxacin (Cipro) 200 mg, 400 mg	400 mg q12h	CrCl 5–29 and HD: 400 mg q24h[a]	Must be combined with metronidazole for anaerobic coverage
Levofloxacin (Levaquin) 250 mg, 500 mg, 750 mg	750 mg q24h	CrCl 20–49: 750 mg q48h CrCl 10–19: 750 mg ×1, then 500 mg q48h HD: 750 mg ×1, then 500 mg q48h[a]	ADR: tendonitis/tendon rupture, CNS effects, peripheral neuropathy, hepatotoxicity, crystalluria, photosensitivity, QT prolongation CI: myasthenia gravis, children due to musculoskeletal toxicity

Moxifloxacin (Avelox) 400 mg	400 mg q24h	—
Nitroimidazole		
Metronidazole 250mg, 500mg	500 mg q8h	Give post HD on HD days

Notes:

- Common pathogens in infected necrosis: *Escherichia coli, Klebsiella, Enterococcus, Pseudomonas*
- Routine use of prophylactic antibiotics in severe acute pancreatitis or sterile necrosis is not recommended
- Carbapenems, quinolones, high-dose cephalosporins, and metronidazole penetrate pancreatic necrosis
- Discontinue empiric antibiotics if pancreatic culture negative
- Treatment duration for confirmed infection up to 14 days

ADR, Adverse drug reaction; *CI*, Contraindication; *CNS*, Central nervous system; *CrCl*, Creatinine clearance; *HD*, Hemodialysis; *IV*, Intravenously; *Pcn*, Penicillin; *PSA*, *Pseudomonas aeruginosa*

aGive post HD on HD days
Data from Tenner S, Baillie J, DeWitt J, Vege SS; American College of Gastroenterology. American College of Gastroenterology guideline: management of acute pancreatitis. *Am J Gastroenterol*. 2013;108(9):1400–1415.

- Empiric antibiotics:
  - Cefotaxime (preferred) or ceftriaxone ×5 days (see Table 10.2)
  - Ofloxacin 400 mg orally (PO) twice daily (BID) as an alternative if no previous exposure to quinolones, hepatic encephalopathy (HE), or serum creatinine >3 mg/dL
- Albumin in high-risk patients (blood urea nitrogen >30 mg/dL, serum creatinine >1 mg/dL, or total bilirubin >4 mg/dL): 1.5 g/kg (within 6 h of the diagnosis of SBP) on day 1 then 1 g/kg on day 3
- Prophylactic antibiotics:
  - Cirrhosis and gastrointestinal hemorrhage
    o Ceftriaxone 1 g IV daily ×7 days
    o May transition to norfloxacin 400 mg PO BID if clinically appropriate (not available in U.S.)
  - Long-term prophylaxis if ascitic fluid protein <1.5 g/dL with impaired renal or liver function
    o Trimethoprim/sulfamethoxazole 1 double-strength PO daily
    o Norfloxacin 400 mg PO daily (not available in U.S.)

Ascites

- Cessation of alcohol consumption
- Sodium restriction: 2 g (88 mEq) per day
- Dual diuretics (100 mg:40 mg=spironolactone:furosemide ratio)
  - Spironolactone:
    - Antagonizes sodium retention
    - Risk of hyperkalemia
    - 100 mg PO daily, max 400 mg daily
    - Discontinue if serum creatinine ≥2 mg/dL
  - Furosemide
    - Promotes urinary sodium loss
    - 40 mg PO/IV daily, max 160 mg daily
    - Discontinue if serum creatinine ≥2 mg/dL
- Avoid or use with caution: NSAIDs, β-blockers, angiotensin-converting enzyme inhibitors, and angiotensin receptor blockers

- Midodrine
  - Alpha1 agonist: increases arteriolar and venous tone
  - 2.5 mg PO TID for refractory ascites; titrate to 7.5 mg TID as needed

Hepatorenal syndrome

- Terlipressin (not available in U.S.)
  - Splanchnic vasoconstrictor
  - 1–2 mg IV q4–6h
- Albumin
  - Volume expander
  - 1 g/kg on day 1, then 10–20 g daily or as needed
- Octreotide
  - Decreases splanchnic blood flow
  - 100–200 mcg subcutaneously TID
- Midodrine
  - Combine with octreotide
  - 5 mg PO TID; titrate to 12.5 mg TID as needed
- Norepinephrine
  - Alpha agonist: vasoconstriction
  - Titrated to goal blood pressure (see Table 12.2)

HEPATIC ENCEPHALOPATHY[3]

Definition

A brain dysfunction caused by impaired hepatic function and/or portosystemic shunting.

Severity

- Grade I: euphoria/depression, mild disorientation, slurred speech
- Grade II: lethargy, moderate disorientation
- Grade III: severe disorientation, incoherent speech, somnolent but arousable
- Grade IV: coma

Management

- Avoid medications that can cause sedation or confusion (i.e., benzodiazepines, anticholinergics)

- Correct precipitating causes
  - Gastrointestinal bleeding
  - Infection
  - Hypokalemia and/or metabolic alkalosis
  - Renal failure
  - Hypovolemia
  - Hypoxia
  - Hypoglycemia
  - Constipation
  - Hepatocellular carcinoma
- Decrease serum ammonia
  - Lactulose: drug of choice
    - Eradicates ammoniagenic bacteria and decrease ammonia absorption from the gastrointestinal tract
    - 25 mL q1–2h until two or more bowel movements per day; titrate to two to three bowel movements per day
  - Rifaximin: add-on to lactulose
    - For patients with inadequate response to lactulose ×48 h
    - Reduction of overt HE recurrence: 550 mg BID PO or via nasogastric tube (NG)
    - Treatment of HE: 400 mg PO/NG q8h ×5–10 days
  - Other therapies with limited data
    - IV L-ornithine L-aspartate
    - Neomycin
    - Metronidazole

References

1. Tenner S, Baillie J, DeWitt J, Vege SS; American College of Gastroenterology. American College of Gastroenterology guideline: management of acute pancreatitis. *Am J Gastroenterol.* 2013;108(9):1400–1415.
2. Runyon BA. Introduction to the revised American Association for the Study of Liver Diseases practice guideline: management of adult patients with ascites due to cirrhosis 2012. *Hepatology.* 2013;57(4):1651–1653.
3. Vilstrup H, Amodio P, Bajaj J, et al. Hepatic encephalopathy in chronic liver disease: 2014 practice guideline by the American Association for the Study of Liver Diseases and the European Association for the Study of the Liver. *Hepatology.* 2014;60(2):715–735.

Infectious
Diseases

10

Abdominal Infections

This chapter will review the guidelines by the Infectious Diseases Society of America (IDSA).

Note: Empiric antibiotics should be tailored based on local pathogen prevalence and antibiotic susceptibility, pathogen-specific risk factors, and previous pathogens and antibiotic exposure. Once final culture and susceptibility results become available, empiric antibiotics should be optimized according to the identified pathogen(s) and susceptibility.

COMPLICATED INTRA-ABDOMINAL INFECTION[1]

Definition

IDSA and Surgical Infection Society define complicated intra-abdominal infection as infection extending beyond the hollow viscus of origin into the peritoneal space that is associated with abscess formation or peritonitis.

Risk Factors for Source Control Failure

- Delay in treatment (>24 h)
- High severity of illness (Acute Physiology and Chronic Health Evaluation II score ≥15)
- Age >70 years
- Medical comorbidity
- Degree of organ dysfunction

- Low albumin
- Poor nutritional status
- Degree of peritoneal involvement or diffuse peritonitis
- Inability to achieve adequate debridement or drainage
- Malignancy

Pathogens in Order of Prevalence

- *Escherichia coli*
- *Bacteroides* species
- *Streptococcus* species
- *Clostridium* species
- *Peptostreptococcus* species, *Eubacterium* species
- *Klebsiella* species, *Pseudomonas aeruginosa*
- *Prevotella* species, *Enterococcus faecalis*

Treatment

- Antibiotic regimen (Table 10.1)
- Antibiotic dosing (Table 10.2)

CLOSTRIDIUM DIFFICILE INFECTION (CDI)[3]

Definitions

CDI is defined as the presence of symptoms (e.g., diarrhea) and a positive stool for *C. difficile* toxin, toxigenic *C. difficile* (e.g., DNA amplication detecting toxin-coding genes), or pseudomembranous colitis on endoscopy or histopathology.

Initial Episode of CDI

A new primary episode of symptom onset (no symptom with positive assay result within the previous 8 weeks) and positive assay result (e.g., toxin enzyme immunoassay or nucleic acid amplification test).

Recurrent Episode of CDI

An episode of symptom onset and positive assay result following an episode with positive result in the previous 2–8 weeks.

Table 10.1 Empiric Antibiotic Therapy for Complicated Intra-Abdominal Infection

TYPE OF INFECTION	ANTIBIOTIC REGIMEN
Community-Acquired Extra-Biliary Intra-Abdominal Infection	
Mild-moderate severity	Cefoxitin Ertapenem Moxifloxacin Tigecycline Ticarcillin-clavulanic acid (unavailable in U.S.) Cefazolin + metronidazole Cefuroxime + metronidazole Ceftriaxone + metronidazole Cefotaxime + metronidazole Ciprofloxacin[a] + metronidazole Levofloxacin[a] + metronidazole
High severity	Imipenem-cilastatin Meropenem Doripenem Piperacillin-tazobactam Cefepime + metronidazole Ceftazidime + metronidazole Ciprofloxacin[a] + metronidazole Levofloxacin[a] + metronidazole
Biliary Intra-Abdominal Infection	
Community-acquired acute cholecystitis of mild to moderate severity	Cefazolin Cefuroxime Ceftriaxone
Community-acquired acute cholecystitis of high severity or acute cholangitis following bilio-enteric anastomosis	Imipenem-cilastatin Meropenem Doripenem Piperacillin-tazobactam Cefepime + metronidazole Ciprofloxacin[a] + metronidazole Levofloxacin[a] + metronidazole
Health care–associated biliary infection	Vancomycin plus one of the following: • Imipenem-cilastatin • Meropenem • Doripenem

Continued

Table 10.1 Empiric Antibiotic Therapy for Complicated Intra-Abdominal Infection—cont'd

TYPE OF INFECTION	ANTIBIOTIC REGIMEN
	• Piperacillin-tazobactam • Cefepime + metronidazole • Ciprofloxacin[a] + metronidazole • Levofloxacin[a] + metronidazole
Health Care–Associated Intra-Abdominal Infection	
<20% resistant *Pseudomonas aeruginosa*, ESBL-producing *Enterobacteriaceae*, *Acinetobacter*, or other MDR GNB	Imipenem-cilastatin Meropenem Doripenem Piperacillin-tazobactam Cefepime + metronidazole Ceftazidime + metronidazole
ESBL-producing *Enterobacteriaceae*, *Pseudomonas aeruginosa* >20% resistant to ceftazidime	Imipenem-cilastatin Meropenem Doripenem Piperacillin-tazobactam Aminoglycoside
MRSA	Vancomycin

ESBL, Extended-spectrum β-lactamase; *GNB*, Gram-negative bacilli; *MDR*, Multidrug resistant; *MRSA*, Methicillin-resistant *Staphylococcus aureus*
[a]Recommend reviewing local population susceptibility reports given increasing resistance of *Escherichia coli* to fluoroquinolones
Adapted from Solomkin JS, Mazuski JE, Bradley JS, et al. Diagnosis and management of complicated intra-abdominal infection in adults and children: guidelines by the Surgical Infection Society and the Infectious Diseases Society of America. *Clin Infect Dis.* 2010;50(12): 133–164.

Nonsevere CDI

White blood cell count (WBC) ≤15,000 cells/mL and serum creatinine <1.5 mg/dL.

Severe CDI

WBC >15,000 cells/mL and/or serum creatinine ≥1.5 mg/dL.

Fulminant CDI

Hypotension, shock, ileus, or megacolon.

Table 10.2 Antibiotic Dosing for Complicated Intra-Abdominal Infection

ANTIBIOTIC	STANDARD DOSE (IV)	RENAL DOSING	COMMENTS
B-Lactam/β-Lactamase Inhibitor Combination			
Piperacillin-tazobactam	Non-PSA: 3.375 g q6h PSA: 4.5 g q6h	Non-PSA: CrCl 20–40: 2.25 g q6h CrCl <20: 2.25 g q8h HD: 2.25 g q12h[a] PSA: CrCl 20–40: 3.375 g q6h CrCl <20: 2.25 g q6h HD: 2.25 g q8h[a]	Off-label extended infusion: 3.375–4.5 g ×1 over 30 min, followed 4 h later by 4 h infusion q8h
Carbapenems (Cross-Sensitivity With PCN Allergy)			
Doripenem	500 mg q8h	CrCl 30–50: 250 mg q8h CrCl 11–29: 250 mg q12h HD: 250 mg q24h[a]; If PSA, 500 mg q12h ×1 then 500 mg 24 h[a]	Similar spectrum of activity as merope- nem except more potent in vitro activity against PSA than meropenem
Ertapenem	1 g q24h	CrCl ≤30 and HD: 500 mg daily	Compared to imipenem or meropenem, less active against PSA, *Acinetobacter*, enterococci, and PCN-resistant *pneumococci*

Continued

Table 10.2 Antibiotic Dosing for Complicated Intra-Abdominal Infection—cont'd

ANTIBIOTIC	STANDARD DOSE (IV)	RENAL DOSING	COMMENTS
Imipenem-cilastatin	500 mg q6h or 1 g q8h	CrCl 60–89: 500 mg q6h CrCl 30–59: 500 mg q8h CrCl 15–29 and HD: 500 mg q12h[a] CrCl <15 without HD: avoid use	Consider decreasing dose in patients <70 kg to prevent seizures
Meropenem	1 g q8h	CrCl 26–50: same dose q12h CrCl 10–25: half dose q12h CrCl <10: half dose q24h HD: 500 mg q24h[a]	Similar spectrum of activity as imipenem; slightly lower risk of seizures than imipenem
Cephalosporins (10% Cross-Sensitivity With PCN Allergy)			
Cefazolin	1–2 g q8h	CrCl 11–34: 50% dose q12h CrCl ≤10 and HD: 50% dose q24h[a]	—
Cefepime	2 g q8–12h	CrCl 30–60: 2 g q12–24h CrCl <30: 1–2 g q24h HD: 0.5–1 g q24h[a]	Risk of seizures in renal insufficiency
Cefotaxime	2 g q8h	CrCl <20: 50% dose q8h HD: 1–2 g q24h[a]	—

Cefoxitin	2 g q6h	CrCl 30–50: 2 g q8–12h CrCl 10–29: 2 g q12–24h CrCl 5–9: 2 g ×1 then 1 g q12–24h CrCl <5 and HD: 2 g ×1 then 1 g q24–48h[a]	—
Ceftazidime	2 g q8h	CrCl 31–50: 2 g q12h CrCl 16–30: 2 g q24h CrCl ≤15 and HD: 1 g q24h[a]	Possible cross-sensitivity between aztreonam and ceftazidime (<5%); avoid aztreonam if history of life-threatening reaction or anaphylaxis to ceftazidime. Other cephalosporins do not have the same risk as ceftazidime
Ceftriaxone	2 g q24h	—	—
Cefuroxime (Zinacef)	1.5 g q8h	CrCl 10–20: 1.5 g q12h CrCl <10 and HD: 1.5 g q24h[a]	—
Ceftazidime 2 g-avibactam 0.5 g (Avycaz 2.5 g)	2.5 g q8h	CrCl 31–50: 1.25 g q8h CrCl 16–30: 0.94 g q12h CrCl 6–15: 0.94 g q24h CrCl ≤5 and HD: 0.94 g q48h[a]	Reserve for MDR PSA, and ESBL- and KPC-producing *Enterobacteriaceae*. Combine with metronidazole
Ceftolozane 1 g-tazobactam 0.5 g (Zerbaxa 1.5 g)	1.5 g q8h	CrCl 30–50: 750 mg q8h CrCl 15–29: 375 mg q8h CrCl <15: not studied HD: 750 mg ×1 then 150 mg q8h[a]	Reserve for MDR PSA and ESBL-producing *Enterobacteriaceae*. Combine with metronidazole

Continued

Table 10.2 Antibiotic Dosing for Complicated Intra-Abdominal Infection—cont'd

ANTIBIOTIC	STANDARD DOSE (IV)	RENAL DOSING	COMMENTS
Glycylcycline			
Tigecycline	100 mg ×1 then 50 mg q12h	—	Increase in all-cause mortality observed in meta-analysis of Phase 3 and 4 clinical trials where greatest differences seen with ventilator-associated pneumonia
Fluoroquinolones			
Ciprofloxacin	400 mg q12h	CrCl 5–29 and HD: 400 mg q24h[a]	ADR: tendonitis/tendon rupture, CNS effects, peripheral neuropathy, hepato-toxicity, crystalluria, photosensitivity, QT prolongation. CI: myasthenia gravis, children due to musculoskeletal toxicity
Levofloxacin	750 mg q24h	CrCl 20–49: 750 mg q48h CrCl 10–19: 750 mg ×1, then 500 mg q48h HD: 750 mg ×1, then 500 mg q48h[a]	"
Moxifloxacin	400 mg q24h	—	"
Nitroimidazole			
Metronidazole	500 mg q8h	Give post HD on HD days	—

Aminoglycosides			
Gentamicin or tobramycin	5–7 mg/kg q24h[b]	CrCl 20–60: 5–7 mg/kg q36–48 h[b] CrCl <20 and HD: 1–2.5 mg/kg LD, then based on level[a,c]	Consult pharmacist for dosing. Goal for once daily dosing: refer to Hartford nomogram[d]. Use adjusted BW for obese
Amikacin	15–20 mg/kg q24h[b]	CrCl 20–60: 15–20 mg/kg q36–48h[b] CrCl <20 and HD: 5 mg/kg LD then based on level[a,c]	"
Monobactam			
Aztreonam	1–2 g q6–8h	CrCl 10–30: 0.5–1 g q6–8h CrCl <10: 250–500 mg q6–8h HD: 1–2 g LD, then 250–500 mg q6–8h[a]	Possible cross-sensitivity between aztreonam and ceftazidime (<5%); see comment on ceftazidime
Glycopeptide			
Vancomycin	15–20 mg/kg q8–12h	CrCl 15–50: 750–1500 mg q24h Max: 2 g/dose CrCl <15: 750–1500 mg based on level[a] HD: 500–1000 mg based on level[a]	Consult pharmacist for dosing Goal trough: 10–15 mcg/mL (15–20 mcg/mL if visceral abscesses) Use actual BW for obese

Notes:
• Surgical management is critical in most intra-abdominal infections
• 4–5 days is the recommended duration who have adequate source control; longer duration is appropriate if inadequate or uncertain source control

Continued

Table 10.2 Antibiotic Dosing for Complicated Intra-Abdominal Infection—cont'd

ANTIBIOTIC	STANDARD DOSE (IV)	RENAL DOSING	COMMENTS
			• Empiric antifungal may be considered for upper gastrointestinal perforations, recurrent bowel perforations, surgically treated pancreatitis, heavy colonization with *Candida* species, or presence of yeast on intra-abdominal cultures
			• *Candida albicans:* Fluconazole IV 800 mg ×1 then 400 mg daily
			• Fluconazole-resistant *Candida* species:
			• Anidulafungin IV 200 mg ×1 then 100 mg daily
			• Caspofungin IV 70 mg ×1 then 50 mg daily
			• Micafungin IV 100 mg daily
			• Antienterococcal therapy: consider in postoperative infection, those who have previously received cephalosporins or other antimicrobial agents selecting for *Enterococcus* species, immunocompromised patients, and those with valvular heart disease or prosthetic intravascular materials
			• Anti-MRSA therapy: consider in patients with MRSA or MDRO risk factors (advanced age, comorbid medical conditions, previous hospitalization/surgery, recent antibiotic agents)

ADR, Adverse drug reaction; *BW,* Body weight; *CI,* Contraindication; *CNS,* Central nervous system; *CrCl,* Creatinine clearance; *ESBL,* Extended-spectrum β-lactamase; *HD,* Hemodialysis; *IV,* Intravenously; *KPC, Klebsiella pneumoniae carbapenemase; LD,* Losing dose; *MDR,* Multidrug resistant; *MDRO,* Multidrug-resistant organism; *MRSA,* Methicillin-resistant *Staphylococcus aureus; PCN,* Penicillin; *PSA: Pseudomonas aeruginosa.*
[a]Give post HD on HD days
[b]Once daily dosing
[c]Conventional dosing
[d]Hartford nomogram: Fig. 10.1
Data from Solomkin JS, Mazuski JE, Bradley JS, et al. Diagnosis and management of complicated intra-abdominal infection in adults and children: guidelines by the Surgical Infection Society and the Infectious Diseases Society of America. *Clin Infect Dis.* 2010;50(2):133–164.

Risk Factors

- Antibiotic therapy
  - All antibiotic classes have been associated with CDI
  - Highest-risk antibiotic classes: fluoroquinolones, third- and fourth-generation cephalosporins, carbapenems, and clindamycin
- Gastric acid-suppressing pharmacotherapy
- Age >65 years
- Hospitalization
- Severe comorbid illness
- Enteral feeding
- Cancer chemotherapy
- Gastrointestinal surgery
- Obesity
- Hematopoietic stem cell transplantation
- Inflammatory bowel disease
- Cirrhosis

Treatment (Table 10.3)

Table 10.3 Treatment of *Clostridium Difficile* Infection

EPISODE AND ILLNESS CATEGORY	TREATMENT
Initial episode, nonsevere CDI	Vancomycin 125 mg PO QID for 10 days, OR Fidaxomicin 200 mg PO BID for 10 days Alternate if above agents are unavailable: metronidazole 500 mg PO TID 10 days
Initial episode, severe CDI	Vancomycin 125 mg PO QID for 10 days, OR Fidaxomicin 200 mg PO BID for 10 days
Initial episode, fulminant CDI	Vancomycin 500 mg PO/NG QID + metronidazole 500 mg IV q8h If ileus, replace PO/NG vancomycin with rectal instillation of vancomycin 500 mg in 0.9% sodium chloride (100–500 mL) via retention enema for 1 h q6h

Continued

Table 10.3 Treatment of Clostridium Difficile Infection—cont'd

EPISODE AND ILLNESS CATEGORY	TREATMENT
First recurrence	If metronidazole was used for the initial episode: vancomycin 125 mg PO QID for 10 days If vancomycin was used for the initial episode: fidaxomicin 200 mg PO BID for 10 days If a standard regimen was used for the initial episode: prolonged tapered and pulsed vancomycin 125 mg PO QID for 10–14 days, BID for 1 week, daily for 1 week, then every 2–3 days for 2–8 weeks
Second or subsequent recurrence	Prolonged tapered and pulsed vancomycin as above, OR Vancomycin 125 mg PO QID for 10 days followed by rifaximin 400 mg PO TID for 20 days, OR Fidaxomicin 200 mg PO BID for 10 days, OR Fecal microbiota transplantation

Notes:

- PO vancomycin, fidaxomicin, and rifaximin are minimally absorbed
- Vancomycin level monitoring is not necessary for PO/NG/rectal route
- Treatment with concomitant antibiotics other than those given to treat CDI may increase risk of treatment failure or recurrent CDI
- Patients with suspected or proven CDI should be placed on contact precautions
- Hand hygiene with soap and water is more effective than alcohol-based hand sanitization in removing *C. difficile* spores

BID, Twice daily; *CDI, Clostridium difficile* infection; *IV,* Intravenously; *NG,* Nasogastric; *PO,* Orally; *QID,* Four times daily; *TID,* three times daily
Adapted from McDonald LC, Gerding DN, Johnson S, et al. Clinical practice guidelines for *Clostridium difficile* infection in adults and children: 2017 Update by the Infectious Diseases Society of America (IDSA) and Society for Healthcare Epidemiology of America (SHE A). *Clin Infect Dis.* 2018;66(7):e1–e48.

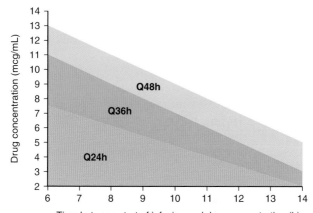

Figure 10.1 The Hartford Nomogram. *Adapted from Nicolau DP, Freeman CD, Belliveau PP, et al. Experience with a once-daily aminoglycoside program administered to 2,184 adult patients. Antimicrob Agents Chemother. 1995;39(3):650–655.*

References

1. Solomkin JS, Mazuski JE, Bradley JS, et al. Diagnosis and management of complicated intra-abdominal infection in adults and children: guidelines by the Surgical Infection Society and the Infectious Diseases Society of America. *Clin Infect Dis.* 2010;50(12):133–164.
2. Nicolau DP, Freeman CD, Belliveau PP, Nightingale CH, Ross JW, Quintiliani R. Experience with a once-daily aminoglycoside program administered to 2,184 adult patients. *Antimicrob Agents Chemother.* 1995;39(3):650–655.
3. McDonald LC, Gerding DN, Johnson S, et al. Clinical practice guidelines for *Clostridium difficile* infection in adults and children: 2017 update by the Infectious Diseases Society of America (IDSA) and Society for Healthcare Epidemiology of America (SHEA). *Clin Infect Dis.* 2018;66(7):e1–e48.

11

Other Infections

This chapter will review the practice guidelines by the Infectious Diseases Society of America (IDSA).

Note: Empiric antibiotics should be tailored based on local pathogen prevalence and antibiotic susceptibility, pathogen-specific risk factors, and previous pathogens and antibiotic exposure. Once final culture and susceptibility results become available, empiric antibiotics should be optimized according to the identified pathogen(s) and susceptibility.

HOSPITAL-ACQUIRED AND VENTILATOR-ASSOCIATED PNEUMONIA[1]

- Definitions:
  - Pneumonia: new lung infiltrate plus clinical evidence of infection such as new fever, purulent sputum, leukocytosis, and oxygen desaturation.
  - Hospital-acquired pneumonia (HAP): a pneumonia developing ≥48 h after hospital admission.
  - Ventilator-associated pneumonia (VAP): a pneumonia developing >48 h after endotracheal intubation.
- Risk factors for multidrug-resistant (MDR) pathogens (Box 11.1)

Box 11.1 Risk Factors for Multidrug-Resistant Pathogens	
HAP	**VAP**
• Previous IV antibiotic therapy within 90 days	• Previous IV antibiotic therapy within 90 days • Septic shock at VAP onset • ARDS preceding VAP • ≥5 days of hospitalization prior to VAP • Acute renal replacement therapy prior to VAP

ARDS, Acute respiratory distress syndrome; *HAP,* Hospital-acquired pneumonia; *IV,* intravenously; *VAP,* Ventilator-associated pneumonia
From Kalil AC, Metersky ML, Klompas M, et al. Management of adults with hospital-acquired and ventilator-associated pneumonia: 2016 clinical practice guidelines by the Infectious Diseases Society of America and the American Thoracic Society. *Clin Infect Dis.* 2016;63(5):e61–e111.

- Pathogens in intensive care unit (ICU) patients:
  - Methicillin-resistant *Staphylococcus aureus* (MRSA)
  - *Pseudomonas aeruginosa* (PSA)
  - Gram-negative bacilli
- Treatment for HAP (Table 11.1)
  - If **NO** risk for MDR pathogens: choose one agent from regimen A that has activity against PSA and methicillin-susceptible *Staphylococcus aureus* (MSSA)
  - If MDR pathogens suspected: choose one agent each from regimen A and B with activity against PSA and one agent from regimen C with activity against MRSA
- Treatment for VAP: same therapy as HAP with risk for MDR

COMMUNITY-ASSOCIATED PNEUMONIA[2]

- Definition: IDSA defines pneumonia as new lung infiltrate plus clinical evidence of infection such as new fever, purulent sputum, leukocytosis, and oxygen desaturation.
- Risk factors for drug-resistant pathogens:
  - Previous antibiotic therapy
  - Recent hospitalization
  - Immunosuppression

Table 11.1 Empiric Antimicrobial Therapy for HAP/VAP in ICU

DRUG	STANDARD DOSING (IV)	RENAL DOSING	DIALYSIS	COMMENTS
Regimen A: Antipseudomonal β-Lactam				
Aztreonam (Azactam) 1 g, 2 g	2 g q8h	CrCl 10–30: 1 g q8h CrCl <10: 500 mg q8h	HD: 2 g LD, then 500 mg q8h[a] CRRT: 2 g q12h	Possible cross-sensitivity between aztreonam and ceftazidime (<5%); avoid aztreonam if history of life-threatening reaction or anaphylaxis to ceftazidime. Other cephalosporins do not have the same risk as ceftazidime. Aztreonam and ceftazidime should be combined with vancomycin/linezolid due to lack of or less activity against gram-positive bacteria
Ceftazidime (Fortaz) 500 mg, 1 g, 2 g	2 g q8h	CrCl 31–50: 2 g q12h CrCl 16–30: 2 g q24h CrCl ≤15: 1 g q24h	HD: 1 g q24h[a] CRRT: 2 g q12h	
Cefepime (Maxipime) 1 g, 2 g	2 g q8h	CrCl 30–60: 2 g q12h CrCl <30: 2 g q24h	HD: 1 g q24h[a] CRRT: 1 g q8h or 2 g q12h	Risk of seizures in renal insufficiency
Imipenem (Primaxin) 250 mg, 500 mg	500 mg q6h	CrCl 10–50: 500 mg q8–12h CrCl <10: 250–500 mg q12h	HD: 250–500 mg q12h[a] CRRT: 500 mg q6–8h	Consider reserving for risk of ESBL producing pathogens Cross-sensitivity with PCN allergy Consider decreasing dose in patients <70 kg to prevent seizures

Drug	Dose	CrCl adjustment	HD / CRRT	Comments
Meropenem (Merrem) 500 mg, 1 g	1 g q8h	CrCl 26–50: 1–2 g q12h CrCl 10–25: 0.5–1 g q12h CrCl <10: 0.5–1 g q24h	HD: 500 mg q24h[a] CRRT: 500 mg–1 g q8h	Consider reserving for risk of ESBL producing pathogens Cross sensitivity w/ PCN allergy
Piperacillin-tazobactam (Zosyn) 2.25 g, 3.375 g, 4.5 g	4.5 g q6h	CrCl 20–40: 3.375 g q6h CrCl <20: 2.25 g q6h	HD: 2.25 g q8h[a] CRRT: 3.375 g q6h	Consider extended infusion for critically ill: 4.5 g ×1 over 30 min, followed 4 h later by 4 h infusion q8h
Regimen B: Antipseudomonal Non-β-Lactam				
Amikacin Standardized doses: 250–750 mg (round to nearest 50 mg)	CD: 5–7.5 mg/kg q8h ODD: 15–20 mg/kg q24h	CrCl 20–60: CD: 5–7.5 mg/kg q12–24h[b] ODD: 15–20 mg/kg q36–48h CrCl <20: CD: 5 mg/kg LD then based on level ODD not recommended	HD: 5 mg/kg[a,b] CRRT: 10 mg/kg LD, then 7.5 mg/kg q24–48h[b]	Consult Pharmacist for dosing Goal level (mcg/mL): Amikacin: peak: 25–35; trough: ≤8 Gentamicin/tobramycin: peak: 6–8; trough: ≤1–2 Goal for ODD: refer to Hartford nomogram (Fig. 10.1) Use ideal or adjusted BW for obese ADR: nephrotoxicity and ototoxicity
Gentamicin/ Tobramycin Standardized doses: 60–120 mg (round to nearest 10 mg)	CD: 1–2.5 mg/kg q8–12h ODD: 5–7 mg/kg q24h	CrCl 20–60: CD: 1–2.5 mg/kg q12–24h[b] ODD: 5–7 mg/kg q36–48h CrCl <20: CD: 1–2.5 mg/kg LD, then based on level ODD not recommended	HD: 1.5–2 mg/kg[a,b] CRRT: 1.5–2 mg/kg q24–48h[b]	"

Continued

Table 11.1 Empiric Antimicrobial Therapy for HAP/VAP in ICU—cont'd

DRUG	STANDARD DOSING (IV)	RENAL DOSING	DIALYSIS	COMMENTS
Ciprofloxacin (Cipro) 200 mg, 400 mg	400 mg q8h	CrCl 5–29: 400 mg q24h	HD: 400 mg q24h[a] CRRT: 400 mg q12–24h	CI: myasthenia gravis, children due to musculoskeletal toxicity. ADR: tendonitis/tendon rupture, photosensitivity, peripheral neuropathy, CNS effects, hepatotoxicity, crystalluria, QT prolongation
Levofloxacin (Levaquin) 250 mg, 500 mg, 750 mg	750 mg daily	CrCl 20–49: 750 mg q48h CrCl 10–19: 750 mg ×1 then 500 mg q48h	HD: 750 mg ×1 then 500 mg q48h[a] CRRT: 750 mg ×1 then 250 mg q24h	"
Colistin (Coly-Mycin M) 150 mg	300 mg CBA ×1 then 150 mg CBA q12h	CrCl 20–50: 300 mg CBA ×1 then 150 mg CBA q24h CrCl <20: 300 mg CBA ×1 then 150 mg CBA q48h	HD: 1.5 mg CBA/ kg q24–48h[a]	ADR: nephrotoxicity Reserve for carbapenemase-producing GNB IV colistin does not achieve adequate concentrations in the lung; consider concurrent inhaled colistin (150 mg CBA q8h over 60 min) for carbapenemase producers

Polymyxin B 50 mg	2.5 mg/kg ×1 then 1.25–1.5 mg/kg q12h	CrCl 30–80: 2.5 mg/kg ×1 then 1–1.5 mg/kg q24h; CrCl <30: 2.5 mg/kg ×1 then 1–1.5 mg/kg q2–3d; Anuric: 2.5 mg/kg ×1 then 1 mg/kg q5–7d	HD: 25 mg IM q24h	10,000 units = 1 mg; ADR: nephrotoxicity; Reserve for carbapenemase-producing GNB

Regimen C for MRSA

Vancomycin (Vancocin) Standardized doses: 0.5–2 g (round to nearest 250 mg)	15–20 mg/kg q8–12h; Consider 25–30 mg/kg LD; Max: 2 g/dose	CrCl 15–50: 750–1500 mg q24h; CrCl <15: 750–1500 mg[b]	HD: 500–1000 mg[a,b]; CRRT: 15–25 mg/kg LD, then 1 g q24–48h[b]	Consult pharmacist for dosing; Goal trough: 15–20 mcg/mL; Use actual BW
Linezolid (Zyvox) 600 mg	600 mg q12h[a]	No change	No change	DDI: discontinue SSRI 2 weeks before linezolid to reduce risk of serotonin syndrome and/or toxicity

Continued

Table 11.1 Empiric Antimicrobial Therapy for HAP/VAP in ICU—cont'd

DRUG	STANDARD DOSING (IV)	RENAL DOSING	DIALYSIS	COMMENTS
Telavancin (Vibativ) 750 mg	10 mg/kg q24h	CrCl 30–50: 7.5 mg/kg q24h CrCl 10–29: 10 mg/kg q48h CrCl <10: not studied	HD/CRRT: not studied	FDA approval for HAP/VAP caused by *Staphylococcus aureus* only Reserve for failure/intolerance to vancomycin/linezolid
New Antimicrobial				
Ceftolozane 1 g-tazobactam 0.5 g (Zerbaxa 1.5 g)	3 g q8h	CrCl 30–50: 1.5 g q8h CrCl 15–29: 750 mg q8h CrCl <15 not on HD: not studied	ESRD on HD: 2.25 g ×1 then 450 mg q8h[a]	Reserve for MDR *Pseudomonas aeruginosa*

Notes:

- If aztreonam replaced by a β-lactam for penicillin allergy, include coverage for MSSA
- For HAP and VAP, a 7-day antibiotic therapy is recommended
- Fluoroquinolones and broad-spectrum cephalosporins have highest risk of C. difficile infection
- Vancomycin and piperacillin-tazobactam combination has been associated with acute kidney injury
- Daptomycin should not be used for HAP/VAP due to inactivation by surfactant and inadequate concentrations in the respiratory track
- Ceftaroline has activity against MRSA, however, only approved by FDA for CAP caused by MSSA or Streptococcus pneumoniae
- Tigecycline has activity against MRSA, however, only approved by FDA for CAP caused by Streptococcus pneumoniae; meta-analysis of Phase 3 and 4 trials demonstrated higher risk of mortality in tigecycline treated patients with VAP
- Among carbapenems, doripenem is not approved by FDA for pneumonia and should not be used

ADR, Adverse drug reaction; *BW*, Body weight; *CAP*, Community-acquired pneumonia; *CBA*, Colistin base activity; *CD*, Conventional dosing; *CI*, Contraindication; *CNS*, Central nervous system; *CrCl*, Creatinine clearance; *CRRT*, Continuous renal replacement therapy; *DDI*, Drug-drug interaction; *ESBL*, Extended-spectrum β-lactamase; *ESRD*, End-stage renal disease; *FDA*, Food and Drug Administration; *GNB*, Gram-negative bacilli; *HAP*, Hospital-acquired pneumonia; *HD*, Hemodialysis; *ICU*, Intensive care unit; *IM*, Intramuscularly; *IV*, Intravenously; *LD*, Losing dose; *MRSA*, Methicillin resistant *Staphylococcus aureus*; *MSSA*, Methicillin-susceptible *Staphylococcus aureus*; *ODD*, Once-daily dosing; *PCN*, penicillin; *SSRI*, Selective serotonin-reuptake inhibitor; *VAP*, Ventilator-associated pneumonia

^aGive post HD on HD days
^bBased on level

Drugs without brand names are denoted by generic name only
Data from Kalil AC, Metersky ML, Klompas M, et al. Management of adults with hospital-acquired and ventilator-associated pneumonia: 2016 clinical practice guidelines by the Infectious Diseases Society of America and the American Thoracic Society. *Clin Infect Dis.* 2016;63(5):e61-em.

- Pulmonary comorbidity (cystic fibrosis, bronchiectasis, frequent glucocorticoid/antibiotic use in chronic obstructive pulmonary disease)
- Aspiration
- Medical comorbidities (diabetes, alcoholism)
- Pathogens in ICU patients:
  - *Streptococcus pneumoniae* (most common)
  - *Staphylococcus aureus*
  - *Legionella species*
  - Gram-negative bacilli
  - *Haemophilus influenzae*
- Treatment (Table 11.2)
  - If **NO** risk for PSA or MRSA: β-lactam plus azithromycin or levofloxacin or moxifloxacin
  - If PSA suspected: antipneumococcal, antipseudomonal β-lactam + one of the following
    - Ciprofloxacin or levofloxacin
    - Aminoglycoside + azithromycin
    - Aminoglycoside + levofloxacin or moxifloxacin
  - If community-acquired MRSA suspected: add vancomycin or linezolid
  - If penicillin allergy: replace a β-lactam with aztreonam and a respiratory fluoroquinolone

INFLUENZA[3]

- Definition: IDSA defines influenza as an acute respiratory illness caused by seasonal influenza A or B viruses.
- Risk factors for complications from influenza:
  - Age <5 years and ≥65 years
  - Chronic pulmonary, cardiovascular, renal, hepatic, hematologic, or metabolic disorders or neurologic and neurodevelopment conditions
  - Immunosuppression
  - Pregnancy or 2 weeks postpartum
  - Children ≤18 years on long-term aspirin
  - American Indians/Alaska Natives

Table 11.2 Empiric Antimicrobial Therapy for CAP in ICU

DRUG	STANDARD DOSING (IV)	RENAL DOSING	DIALYSIS	COMMENTS
β-Lactams				
Cefotaxime (Claforan) 1 g, 2 g	1–2 g q8h	CrCl <20: 50% dose q8h	HD: 1–2 g q24h[a] CRRT: 1–2 g q8h	10% cross-sensitivity with PCN allergy
Ceftaroline (Teflaro) 400 mg, 600 mg	600 mg q12h	CrCl 31–50: 400 mg q12h CrCl 15–30: 300 mg q12h CrCl <15: 200 mg q12h	HD: 200 mg q12h[a] CRRT: 200 mg q12h	"
Ceftriaxone (Rocephin) 1 g, 2 g	1–2 g daily[a]	No change	No change	"
Ampicillin-sulbactam (Unasyn) 1.5 g, 3 g	3 g q6h	CrCl 15–29: 3 g q12h CrCl <15: 3 g q24h	HD: 3 g q12–24h[a] CRRT: 3 g q8h	—
Ertapenem (Invanz) 1 g	1 g daily	CrCl ≤30: 500 mg daily	HD: 500 mg daily[a]	Cross-sensitivity with PCN allergy
Azithromycin and Quinolones				
Azithromycin (Zithromax) 500 mg	500 mg daily	No change	No change	ADR: QT prolongation, hepato-toxicity

Continued

Table 11.2 Empiric Antimicrobial Therapy for CAP in ICU—cont'd

DRUG	STANDARD DOSING (IV)	RENAL DOSING	DIALYSIS	COMMENTS
Ciprofloxacin (Cipro) 200 mg, 400 mg	400 mg q8h	CrCl 5–29: 400 mg q24h	HD: 400 mg q24h[a] CRRT: 400 mg q12–24h	CI: myasthenia gravis, children due to musculoskeletal toxicity. ADR: tendonitis/tendon rupture, peripheral neuropathy, CNS effects, photosensitivity, hepatoxicity, crystalluria, QT prolongation
Levofloxacin (Levaquin) 250 mg, 500 mg, 750 mg	750 mg daily	CrCl 20–49: 750 mg q48h CrCl 10–19: 750 mg ×1 then 500 mg q48h	HD: 750 mg ×1 then 500 mg q48h[a] CRRT: 750 mg ×1 then 250 mg q24h	"
Moxifloxacin (Avelox) 400 mg	400 mg daily	No change	No change	"
Antipneumococcal, Antipseudomonal β-Lactams				
Piperacillin-tazobactam (Zosyn) 2.25 g, 3.375 g, 4.5 g	4.5 g q6h	CrCl 20–40: 3.375 g q6h CrCl <20: 2.25 g q6h	HD: 2.25 g q8h[a] CRRT: 3.375 g q6h	Off-label extended infusion: 3.375–4.5 g ×1 over 30 min, followed 4 h later by 4 h infusion q8h

Drug	Dose	Renal dosing	HD/CRRT	Comments
Cefepime (Maxipime) 1 g, 2 g	2 g q8h	CrCl 30–60: 2 g q12h CrCl <30: 2 g q24h	HD: 1 g q24h[a] CRRT: 1 g q8h or 2 g q12h	Risk of seizures in renal insufficiency
Ceftazidime (Fortaz) 500 mg, 1 g, 2 g	2 g q8h	CrCl 31–50: 2 g q12h CrCl 16–30: 2 g q24h CrCl ≤15: 1 g q24h	HD: 1 g q24h[a] CRRT: 2 g q12h	Possible cross-sensitivity between aztreonam and ceftazidime (<5%): see Table 11.1 for detail
Imipenem (Primaxin) 250 mg, 500 mg	500 mg q6h	CrCl 10–50: 500 mg q8–12h CrCl <10: 250–500 mg q12h	HD: 250–500 mg q12h[a] CRRT: 500 mg q6–8h	Cross-sensitivity with PCN allergy. Consider decreasing dose in patients <70 kg to prevent seizures
Meropenem (Merrem) 500 mg, 1 g	1 g q8h	CrCl 26–50: 1–2 g q12h CrCl 10–25: 500 mg–1 g q12h CrCl <10: 500 mg–1 g q24h	HD: 500 mg q24h[a] CRRT: 500 mg–1 g q8h	Cross-sensitivity with PCN allergy

Continued

Table 11.2 Empiric Antimicrobial Therapy for CAP in ICU—cont'd

DRUG	STANDARD DOSING (IV)	RENAL DOSING	DIALYSIS	COMMENTS
Aminoglycosides				
Amikacin Standardized doses: 250–750 mg (round to nearest 50 mg)	CD: 5–7.5 mg/kg q8h ODD: 15–20 mg/kg q24h	CrCl 20–60: CD: 5–7.5 mg/kg q12–24h[b] ODD: 15–20 mg/kg q36–48h CrCl <20: CD: 5 mg/kg load then based on level ODD not recommended	HD: 5 mg/kg[a,b] CRRT: LD, then 7.5 mg/kg q24–48h[b]	Consult pharmacist for dosing Goal level (mcg/mL): Amikacin: peak: 25–35; trough: ≤8 Gentamicin/tobramycin: peak: 6–8; trough: ≤1–2 Goal for ODD: refer to Hartford nomogram (Fig. 10.1) Use ideal or adjusted BW for obese ADR: nephrotoxicity and ototoxicity
Gentamicin/Tobramycin Standardized doses: 60–120 mg (round to nearest 10 mg)	CD: 1–2.5 mg/kg q8–12h ODD: 5–7 mg/kg q24h	CrCl 20–60: CD: 1–2.5 mg/kg q12–24h[b] ODD: 5–7 mg/kg q36–48h CrCl <20: CD: 1–2.5 mg/kg load, then based on level ODD not recommended	HD: 1.5–2 mg/kg[a,b] CRRT: 1.5–2 mg/kg q24–48h[b]	"

Antibiotics for CA-MRSA

Vancomycin (Vancocin) Standardized doses: 0.5–2 g (round to nearest 250 mg)	15–20 mg/kg q8–12h Consider 25–30 mg/kg LD Max: 2 g/dose	CrCl 15–50: 750–1500 mg q24h CrCl <15: 750–1500 mg[b]	HD: 500–1000 mg[a,b] CRRT: 15–25 mg/kg load, then 1 g q24–48h[b]	Consult pharmacist for dosing Goal trough: 15–20 mcg/mL Use actual BW
Linezolid (Zyvox) 600 mg	600 mg q12h	No change	No change Give post HD on HD days	DDI: discontinue SSRI 2 weeks before linezolid to reduce risk of serotonin syndrome or toxicity

Monobactam for Penicillin-Allergy

Aztreonam (Azactam) 1 g, 2 g	2 g q8h	CrCl 10–30: 1 g q8h CrCl <10: 500 mg q8h	HD: 2 g LD, then 500 mg q8h[a] CRRT: 2 g q12h	If life-threatening or anaphylactic reaction to penicillin/cephalosporins, replace aztreonam with levofloxacin + AG

New Antimicrobials

Omadacycline (Nuzyra) 100 mg IV 150 mg PO	200 mg IV ×1 then 100 mg IV or 300 mg PO q24h	No change	No change	Broad spectrum of activity against atypical CAP pathogens, MRSA, many GNR, and anaerobes, but NO coverage against PSA

Continued

Table 11.2 Empiric Antimicrobial Therapy for CAP in ICU—cont'd

DRUG	STANDARD DOSING (IV)	RENAL DOSING	DIALYSIS	COMMENTS
Delafloxacin (Baxdela)		Activity against MRSA and PSA, but not FDA approved for the treatment of respiratory tract infections		
Lefamulin		Pending FDA approval: a semisynthetic pleuromutilin antibiotic with narrow spectrum of activity against MRSA, *Streptococcus pneumoniae*, *Haemophilus influenza*, *Moraxella catarrhalis*, and atypical CAP pathogens		

Notes:

- Minimum 5 days is the recommended duration with those who have resolution of symptoms
- A longer duration of treatment may be necessary if empiric therapy was not active against the identified pathogen or if concomitant extrapulmonary infection such as meningitis or endocarditis
- For patients with QT prolongation, doxycycline may replace macrolides and fluoroquinolones
- Vancomycin and piperacillin-tazobactam combination has been associated with acute kidney injury

ADR, Adverse drug reaction; AG, Aminoglycoside; BW, Body weight; CA, Community acquired; CAP, Community-acquired pneumonia; CI, Contraindication; CNS, Central nervous System; CD, Conventional dosing; CrCl, Creatinine clearance; CRRT, Continuous renal replacement therapy; DDI, Drug-drug interaction; FDA, Food and drug administration; GNR, gram-negative rods; HD, Hemodialysis; ICU, Intensive care unit; IV, Intravenously; LD, Loading dose; MRSA, Methicillin-resistant Staphylococcus aureus; ODD, Once daily dosing; PCN, Penicillin; PO, Take orally; PSA, Pseudomonas aeruginosa; SSRI, Selective serotonin-reuptake inhibitors

^aGive post HD on HD days

^bBased on level

Data from Mandell LA, Wunderink RG, Anzueto A, et al.; Infectious Diseases Society of America; American Thoracic Society. Infectious Diseases Society of America/American Thoracic Society consensus guidelines on the management of community-acquired pneumonia in adults. *Clin Infect Dis.* 2007;44(S2):S27–S72.

- Obesity (body mass index $\geq 40 \ kg/m^2$)
- Residents of nursing homes and long-term care facilities
- Pharmacologic management of influenza (Table 11.3)

INTRAVASCULAR CATHETER-RELATED INFECTIONS[4]

- Definitions:
  - The Centers for Disease Control and Prevention (CDC) defines central line-associated bloodstream infections as a primary laboratory-confirmed bloodstream infection occurring >2 days from catheter placement and no later than 1 day after catheter removal.
  - IDSA defines catheter-related bloodstream infection as minimally bacteremia or fungemia in a patient with an intravascular device and more than one positive blood culture from a peripheral vein, clinical manifestation of infection, and no apparent source for bloodstream infection other than the catheter.
- Risk factors:
  - Total parenteral nutrition
  - Prolonged use of broad-spectrum antibiotics
  - Hematologic malignancy
  - Bone marrow or solid-organ transplant
  - Femoral catheter
  - Colonization of *Candida* species at multiple sites
- Pathogens
  - Coagulase-negative staphylococci (*Staphylococcus epidermidis*): most common
  - *Staphylococcus aureus*
  - *Candida* species
  - Enteric gram-negative bacilli (*Escherichia coli*, *Klebsiella* species, *Enterobacter* species)
- Treatment
  - Catheter management (remove, salvage, or exchange)
  - Antibiotics (Table 11.4)
    - Empiric: vancomycin for MRSA
    - Neutropenia: choose an agent against *Pseudomonas aeruginosa*

Table 11.3 Influenza-Specific Pharmacotherapy

DRUG	INFLUENZA ACTIVITY	STANDARD DOSING	RENAL DOSING	COMMENTS
Selective Inhibitor of Influenza Cap-Dependent Endonuclease				
Baloxavir (Xofluza)	A and B	Treatment (PO): a single dose within 48 h of influenza symptoms 40–79 kg: 40 mg ≥80 kg: 80 mg	No change	New agent ADR: diarrhea, nasopharyngitis
Neuraminidase Inhibitors: Drug of Choice				
Oseltamivir (Tamiflu)	A and B	Treatment (PO/NG): 75 mg BID ×5 days 150 mg BID has been used for severe influenza Prophylaxis (PO/NG): 75 mg daily	CrCl 30–60: 30 mg BID CrCl 10–30: 30 mg daily HD: 30 mg ×1 then 30 mg after every HD ×5 days[a] CRRT: 30 mg daily ×5 days or 75 mg q48h ×5 days	ADR: headache, nausea, vomiting, delirium Preferred in severe influenza Consider longer duration of therapy for who remain severely ill after 5 days of therapy

Peramivir (Rapivab)	A and B; limited coverage for B	Treatment (IV): Uncomplicated: 600 mg ×1 Complicated: 600 mg daily ×5–10 days if hospitalized, high risk	Uncomplicated: CrCl 30–49: 200 mg ×1 CrCl <30: 100 mg ×1 Complicated: CrCl 31–49: 150 mg daily CrCl 10–30: 100 mg daily CrCl <10: 100 mg ×1 then 15 mg daily ESRD on HD: 100 mg ×1 then 100 mg 2 h after HD	ADR: diarrhea, neutropenia, hypersensitivity reactions, delirium
Zanamivir (Relenza)	A and B	Treatment (oral inh): two inhalations (10 mg) BID ×5 days Prophylaxis (oral inh): two inhalations (10 mg) daily	No change	ADR: allergic reactions, nausea, diarrhea, headache, decline in respiratory function in patients with asthma/COPD, dizziness, bronchospasm Avoid in chronic lung disease or severe influenza Incompatible with mechanical ventilator circuit

Continued

Table 11.3 Influenza-Specific Pharmacotherapy—cont'd

DRUG	INFLUENZA ACTIVITY	STANDARD DOSING	RENAL DOSING	COMMENTS
Adamantanes: Not Recommended Due To High Resistance to Influenza A				
Amantadine (Symmetrel)	A only	Treatment/prophylaxis: 200 mg daily or 100 mg BID	CrCl 30–50: 200 mg ×1 then 100 mg daily CrCl 15–29: 200 mg ×1 then 100 mg QOD CrCl <15 and HD: 200 mg q7d CRRT: 100 mg daily or QOD	ADR: presyncope/syncope, orthostatic hypotension, falling, peripheral edema, illusion, dizziness, delusions, lower seizure threshold, insomnia, hallucination, paranoia, anticholinergic effects
Rimantadine (Flumadine)	A only	Treatment/prophylaxis: 100 mg BID ×5–7 days	CrCl <30: 100 mg daily	ADR: anticholinergic effects, dizziness, vomiting, nausea

Notes:
- If indicated, initiate antiviral therapy promptly; most effective if started within 48 h of symptom onset
- Treatment not recommended for uncomplicated influenza presenting >48 h of symptoms onset

ADR, Adverse drug reaction; *BID,* Twice daily; *COPD,* Chronic obstructive pulmonary disease; *ESRD,* End-stage renal disease; *HD,* Hemodialysis; *inh,* Inhalation; *IV,* Intravenously; *NG,* Via nasogastric tube; *PO,* Orally; *QOD,* Every other day

^aGive post HD on HD days

Data from Uyeki TM, Bernstein HH, Bradley JS, et al. Clinical practice guidelines by the Infectious Diseases Society of America: 2018 Update on diagnosis, treatment, chemoprophylaxis, and institutional outbreak management of seasonal influenzaa. *Clin Infect Dis.* 2018; 68(6):e1-e47.

Table 11.4 Pathogen-Specific Antimicrobial Therapy for IV CRBSI

PATHOGEN	PREFERRED ANTIBIOTIC (IV)	ALTERNATIVE ANTIBIOTIC (IV)	RENAL DOSING
Gram-Positive Cocci			
Staphylococcus aureus			
Methicillin susceptible	Nafcillin 2 g q4h Oxacillin 2 g q4h	Cefazolin 2 g q8h Vancomycin[a]	Cefazolin: CrCl 11–34: 50% dose q12h CrCl ≤10 and HD: 50% q24h[b] CRRT: 2 g q12h[b]
Methicillin resistant	Vancomycin[a]	Daptomycin 6–8 mg/kg q24h Linezolid[a] TMP-SMX 3–5 mg/kg q8h Vancomycin[b] + rifampin 300–600 mg q12h or genta- micin 1 mg/kg q8h[c]	Daptomycin: CrCl<30 and HD: 6 mg/kg q48h[b] CRRT: 8 mg/kg q48h TMP-SMX: CrCl 10–30: 3–5 mg/kg q12h CrCl <10 and HD: 3–5 mg/kg q24h[b] CRRT: 3–5 mg/kg q12h
Coagulase-Negative *Staphylococci* (CoNS)			
Methicillin susceptible	Nafcillin 2 g q4h Oxacillin 2 g q4h	Cefazolin 2 g q8h[d] Vancomycin[a] TMP-SMX 3–5 mg/kg q8h	Cefazolin: see above TMP-SMX: see above

Continued

Table 11.4 Pathogen-Specific Antimicrobial Therapy for IV CRBSI—cont'd

PATHOGEN	PREFERRED ANTIBIOTIC (IV)	ALTERNATIVE ANTIBIOTIC (IV)	RENAL DOSING
Methicillin resistant	Vancomycin[a]	Daptomycin 6 mg/kg q24h Linezolid[a] Quinupristin/dalfopristin 7.5 mg/kg q8h	Daptomycin: see above
Enterococcus faecalis/faecium			
Ampicillin susceptible	Ampicillin 2 g q4–6h ± gentamicin 1 mg/kg q8h[c]	Vancomycin[a]	Ampicillin: CrCl 10–50: 2 g q6–12h CrCl <10 and HD: 2 g q12–24h[b] CRRT: 2 g q8h
Ampicillin resistant, vancomycin susceptible	Vancomycin[a] ± gentamicin 1 mg/kg q8h[c]	Daptomycin 6 mg/kg q24h Linezolid[a]	Daptomycin: see above
Ampicillin/vancomycin resistant	Daptomycin 6 mg/kg q24h Linezolid[a]	Quinupristin/dalfopristin 7.5 mg/kg q8h (only effective against *E. faecium*)	Daptomycin: see above

Gram-Negative Bacilli

Escherichia coli and Klebsiella Species

ESBL negative	Ceftriaxone 1–2 g q24h[e]	Ciprofloxacin 400 mg q12h Aztreonam[a]	Ciprofloxacin: CrCl 5–29 and HD: 400 mg q24h[b] CRRT: 400 mg q12–24h
ESBL positive	Ertapenem[f] Imipenem[a] Meropenem[a] Doripenem 500 mg q8h	Ciprofloxacin 400 mg q12h Aztreonam[a]	Doripenem: CrCl 30–50: 250 mg q8h CrCl 11–29: 250 mg q12h HD: 250 mg q24h[b] Ciprofloxacin: see above
Enterobacter species and Serratia marcescens	Ertapenem[f] Imipenem[a] Meropenem[a]	Cefepime[a] Ciprofloxacin 400 mg q12h	Ciprofloxacin: see above
Acinetobacter species	Ampicillin/sulbactam[f] Imipenem[a] Meropenem[a]	N/A	—
Stenotrophomonas maltophilia	TMP-SMX 3–5 mg/kg q8h	N/A	TMP-SMX: see above

Continued

Table 11.4 Pathogen-Specific Antimicrobial Therapy for IV CRBSI—contd

PATHOGEN	PREFERRED ANTIBIOTIC (IV)	ALTERNATIVE ANTIBIOTIC (IV)	RENAL DOSING
Pseudomonas aeruginosa	Cefepime[a,g] Imipenem[a] Meropenem[a] Piperacillin-tazobactam[a] Amikacin[a] Tobramycin[a]	N/A	—
Burkholderia cepacia	TMP-SMX 3–5 mg/kg q8h Imipenem[a] Meropenem[a]	N/A	TMP-SMX: see above
Fungi			
***Candida* species**	Caspofungin 70 mg ×1 then 50 mg q24h Micafungin 100 mg q24h Anidulafungin 200 mg ×1 then 100 mg q24h	Lipid amphotericin B 3–5 mg/kg q24h Fluconazole 400–600 mg q24h	—

Uncommon Pathogens

Corynebacterium jeikeium (group JK)	Vancomycin[a]	Linezolid[a]	—
Chryseobacterium (Flavobacterium) species	Levofloxacin[a]	TMP-SMX 3–5 mg/kg q8h Imipenem[a] Meropenem[a]	TMP-SMX: see above
Ochrobactrum anthropi	TMP-SMX 3–5 mg/kg q8h Ciprofloxacin 400 mg q12h	AG[a] + a carbapenem below Imipenem[a] Meropenem[a] Ertapenem[a] Doripenem 500 mg q8h	TMP-SMX: see above Ciprofloxacin: see above Doripenem: see above
Malassezia furfur	Lipid amphotericin B 3–5 mg/kg q24h	Voriconazole 6 mg/kg q12h ×2 then 4 mg/kg q12h	Voriconazole: CrCl <50: avoid IV voriconazole; consider PO voriconazole 200–300 mg q12h or 3–4 mg/kg q12h

Continued

Table 11.4 Pathogen-Specific Antimicrobial Therapy for IV CRBSI—cont'd

PATHOGEN	PREFERRED ANTIBIOTIC (IV)	ALTERNATIVE ANTIBIOTIC (IV)	RENAL DOSING

Notes:

- Duration of therapy
  - Uncomplicated CRBSI: 14 days
  - Complicated CRBSI (endocarditis; immunosuppression, diabetes, chronic intravascular hardware, positive blood cultures >72 h from start of appropriate therapy, septic thrombus, thrombophlebitis): 4–6 weeks
  - Osteomyelitis: 6–8 weeks
- Transesophageal echocardiogram for *Staphylococcus aureus* bacteremia to rule out infective endocarditis
- Although daptomycin, linezolid, tedizolid, telavancin, dalbavancin, oritavancin, ceftaroline, and quinupristin/dalfopristin have activity against CoNS and MRSA, clinical data are limited
- Lipid formulations of amphotericin B do not adequately concentrate in the urine; use amphotericin B deoxycholate 0.3–0.5 mg/kg q24 if urinary tract infection

---

CrCl, Creatinine clearance; *CRBSI,* Catheter-related bloodstream infection; *CRRT,* Continuous renal replacement therapy; *ESBL,* Extended-spectrum β-lactamase; *HD,* Hemodialysis; *IV,* Intravenous; *N/A,* Not applicable; *TMP-SMX,* Trimethoprim-sulfamethoxazole

aSee Table 11.1 for dosing
bGive post HD on HD days
cConsult pharmacy for dosing
dMay substitute with first generation cephalosporin
eMay substitute with third generation cephalosporin
fSee Table 11.2 for dosing
gMay substitute with fourth generation cephalosporin
Medications without notes/notation do not require renal adjustment

Adapted from Mermel LA, Allon M, Bouza E, et al. Clinical practice guidelines for the diagnosis and management of intravascular catheter-related infection: 2009 update by the Infectious Diseases Society of America. *Clin Infect Dis.* 2009;49:1–45.

CATHETER-ASSOCIATED URINARY TRACT INFECTIONS (CAUTIs)[5]

- Definitions:
  - The CDC defines CAUTI as urinary tract infection (UTI) in which an indwelling urinary catheter was in place for >2 days and attributable to the catheter removed no more than 1 day before infection.
  - IDSA defines CAUTI as the presence of signs/symptoms of UTI with $\geq 10^3$ cfu/mL of one or more bacterial species in urine specimen from a patient whose urethral, suprapubic, or condom catheter currently exists or has been removed within the previous 48 h.
- Risk factor: presence of an indwelling urinary catheter
- Pathogen:
  - *E. coli* (accounts for one-third of CAUTIs)
  - *Klebsiella* spp.; *Proteus* spp.; *Enterobacter* spp.; PSA, *Enterococcus* spp.; MSSA; MRSA; methicillin-resistant *Staphylococcus epidermidis* (MRSE)
  - *Candida* spp. (accounts for up to one-third of CAUTIs)
- Treatment
  - Obtain urinary culture
  - Remove catheter or replace if still indicated
  - Empiric antibiotics (Table 11.5)
  - Duration: 7 days if signs/symptoms resolve within 72 h of antibiotic therapy and up to 14 days if signs/symptoms resolve >72 h

SKIN AND SOFT TISSUE INFECTIONS (SSTIs)[6]

- Management of localized staphylococcal infections (Fig. 11.1)
- Management of surgical site infections (Fig. 11.2)
- Antimicrobial therapy for SSTIs (Table 11.6)
- Antimicrobial therapy for necrotizing infections (Table 11.7)

Table 11.5 Antimicrobial Therapy for CAUTI

DRUG	STANDARD DOSING (IV)	RENAL DOSING	DIALYSIS	COMMENTS
Regimen A: No Risk Factors for Multidrug Resistance				
Ciprofloxacin (Cipro) 200 mg, 400 mg	400 mg IV q12h	CrCl 5–29: 400 mg q24h	HD: 400 mg q24h[a] CRRT: 400 mg IV q12–24h	ADR: tendonitis/tendon rupture, peripheral neuropathy, CNS effects, hepatotoxicity, photosensitivity, crystalluria, QT prolongation Cl: myasthenia gravis, children due to musculoskeletal toxicity Duration: 5 days if not severely ill
Levofloxacin (Levaquin) 250 mg, 500 mg, 750 mg	750 mg IV daily	CrCl 20–49: 750 mg q48h CrCl 10–19: 750 mg ×1, then 500 mg q48h	HD: 750 mg ×1, then 500 mg q48h[a] CRRT: 750 mg ×1, then 250–750 mg q24h	
Ceftriaxone (Rocephin) 1 g, 2 g	1 g IV daily	N/A	Give post HD on HD days	10% cross-sensitivity with PCN allergy

Piperacillin-tazobactam (Zosyn) 2.25 g, 3.375 g, 4.5 g	Non-PSA dose: 3.375 g q6h; PSA dose: 4.5 g q6h	Non-PSA dose: CrCl 20–40: 2.25 g q6h; CrCl <20: 2.25 g q8h; PSA dose: CrCl 20–40: 3.375 g q6h; CrCl <20: 2.25 g q6h	HD: Non-PSA dose: 2.25 g q12h[a]; PSA dose: 2.25 g q8h[a]; CRRT: Non-PSA dose: 2.25 g q6h; PSA dose: 3.375 g q6h	Off-label extended infusion: 3.375–4.5 g ×1 over 30 min, followed 4 h later by 4 h infusion q8h

Regimen B: for Suspected ESBL (Switch Regimen A to B)

Imipenem (Primaxin) 250 mg, 500 mg	500 mg IV q6h	CrCl 10–50: 500 mg q8–12h; CrCl <10: 250–500 mg q12h	HD: 250–500 mg q12h[a]; CRRT: 500 mg q6–8h	Imipenem: consider decreasing dose in patients <70 kg to prevent seizures
Meropenem (Merrem) 500 mg, 1 g	1 g every 8 h	CrCl 26–50: 1 g q12h; CrCl 10–25: 0.5 g q12h; CrCl <10: 0.5 g q24h	HD: 0.5 g q24h; CRRT: 0.5–1 g q8h	Similar spectrum of activity as imipenem; slightly lower risk of seizures than imipenem

Continued

Table 11.5 Antimicrobial Therapy for CAUTI—cont'd

DRUG	STANDARD DOSING (IV)	RENAL DOSING	DIALYSIS	COMMENTS
Doripenem (Doribax) 250 mg, 500 mg	500 mg IV q8h	CrCl 30–50: 250 mg q8h CrCl 11–29: 250 mg q12h	HD: 250 mg q24h[a] If PSA, 500 mg q12h ×1 then 500 mg q24h[a]	Similar spectrum of activity as meropenem except more potent in vitro activity against PSA than meropenem
Regimen C: For Suspected Drug-Resistant Gram-Positive Pathogen (Add to Regimen A or B)				
Vancomycin (Vancocin) Standardized doses: 0.5–2 g (round to nearest 250 mg)	15 mg/kg IV q12h	CrCl 15–50: 750–1500 mg q24h CrCl <15: 750–1500 mg[b]	HD: 500–1000 mg[a,b] CRRT: 15–25 mg/kg ×1, then 1 g q24–48h[b]	Consult pharmacist for dosing Goal trough: 10–15 mcg/mL Use actual BW
Daptomycin (Cubicin) 500 mg	6 mg/kg IV q24h	CrCl <30: 6 mg/kg IV q48h	HD: 6 mg/kg q48h[a] CRRT: 8 mg/kg q48h	Possible myopathy
Linezolid (Zyvox) 600 mg	600 mg IV/PO q12h	No change	Give post HD on HD days	DDI: discontinue SSRI 2 weeks before linezolid to reduce risk of serotonin syndrome/toxicity

Note:

- 7 days is the recommended duration who have prompt resolution of symptoms
- 10–14 days of treatment is recommended for those with a delayed response
- Carbapenems have cross-sensitivity with PCN allergy

ADR, Adverse drug reaction; *BW*, Body weight; *CAUTI*, Catheter-associated urinary tract infection; *CI*, Contraindication; *CNS*, Central nervous system; *CrCl*, Creatinine clearance; *CRRT*, Continuous renal replacement therapy; *DDI*, Drug-drug interaction; *ESBL*, Extended-spectrum β-lactamase; *HD*, Hemodialysis; *IV*, Intravenously; *N/A*, Not applicable; *PCN*, Penicillin; *PSA*, *Pseudomonas aeruginosa*; *SSRI*, Selective serotonin-reuptake inhibitors

^aGive post HD on HD days

^bBased on level

Data from Hooton TM, Bradley SF, Cardenas DD, et al. Diagnosis, prevention, and treatment of catheter-associated urinary tract infection in adults: 2009 international clinical practice guidelines from the Infectious Diseases Society of America. *Clin Infect Dis.* 2010;50(5):625–663.

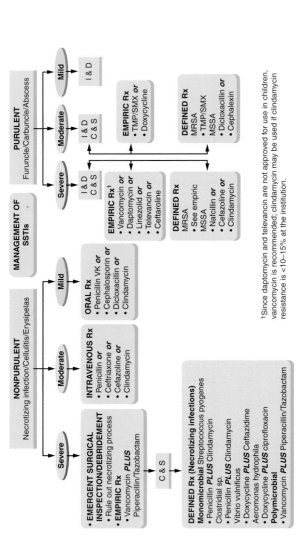

Figure 11.1 Management of Skin and Soft tissue Infections (SSTIs). C & S, Culture and sensitivity; I & D, Incision and drainage; MRSA, Methicillin-resistant Staphylococcus aureus; MSSA, Methicillin-sensitive Staphylococcus aureus; Rx, Treatment; TMP/SMX, Trimethoprim-sulfamethoxazole. From Stevens DL, Bisno AL, Chambers HF, et al. Infectious Diseases Society of America. Practice guidelines for the diagnosis and management of skin and soft tissue infections: 2014 update by the Infectious Diseases Society of America. Clin Infect Dis. 2014;59(2):e10–e52.

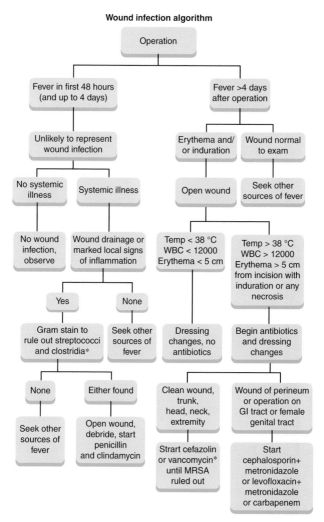

Figure 11.2 Management of Surgical Site Infections (SSIs). *GI,* Gastrointestinal; *MRSA,* Methicillin-resistant *Staphylococcus aureus; WBC,* White blood cell count. *From Stevens DL, Bisno AL, Chambers HF, et al. Infectious Diseases Society of America. Practice guidelines for the diagnosis and management of skin and soft tissue infections: 2014 update by the Infectious Diseases Society of America. Clin Infect Dis. 2014;59(2):e10–e52.*

Table 11.6 Antimicrobial Therapy for SSTIs

	STANDARD DOSING	RENAL DOSING	COMMENTS
Purulent SSTI: *Methicillin-Susceptible Staphylococcus aureus* (MSSA)			
Nafcillin	1–2 g IV q4h	N/A	Antimicrobial of choice; bactericidal activity (applies to nafcillin & oxacillin)
Oxacillin	1–2 g IV q4h	N/A	
Cefazolin	1 g IV q8h	CrCl 11–34: 50% dose q12h CrCl ≤10 and HD: 50% dose q24h[a]	Cross-sensitivity with PCN allergy Bactericidal activity
Clindamycin	600 mg IV q8h or 300–450 mg PO QID	N/A	Use if clindamycin resistance <10–15% Bacteriostatic activity
Dicloxacillin	500 mg PO QID	N/A	Oral agent of choice
Cephalexin	500 mg PO QID	CrCl 30–59: 500 mg BID CrCl 15–29: 250 mg BID CrCl 5–14: 250 mg daily CrCl 1–4: 250 mg q48h HD: 250–500 mg q12–24h[a]	Reserve for mild infection
Doxycycline	100 mg PO BID	N/A	Reserve for mild infection

Minocycline	200 mg PO ×1 then 100 mg PO BID	N/A	Reserve for mild infection
Trimethoprim-sulfamethoxazole	One to two DS tablets PO BID	CrCl 15–30: 50% dose CrCl <15: avoid use	"
Purulent SSTI: *Methicillin-resistant Staphylococcus aureus* (MRSA)			
Vancomycin	15 mg/kg IV q12h[b] Use actual BW Max: 2 g/dose Goal trough: 10–15 mcg/mL	CrCl 15–50: 750–1500 mg q24h CrCl <15: 750–1500 mg based on level HD: 500–1000 mg based on level[a]	Antimicrobial of choice MRSA with vancomycin MIC ≥ 2 mcg/mL may lead to therapeutic failure Bactericidal activity
Daptomycin	4 mg/kg IV q24h	CrCl <30 and HD: 4 mg/kg q48h[a]	Possible myopathy Bactericidal activity
Linezolid	600 mg IV/PO q12h[a]	N/A	Oxazolidinones Bacteriostatic activity High cost and toxicity
Tedizolid	200 mg IV/PO q24h	N/A	"

Continued

Table 11.6 Antimicrobial Therapy for SSTIs—cont'd

	STANDARD DOSING	RENAL DOSING	COMMENTS
Delafloxacin	300 mg IV q12h 450 mg PO q12h	CrCl 15–29: • Oral: N/A • IV: 200 mg q12h CrCl <15 and HD: avoid use	Fluoroquinolone Bactericidal activity
Omadacycline	IV: 200 mg ×1 then 100 mg q24h PO: 450 mg ×1 then 300 mg PO q24h	N/A	Tetracycline; bacteriostatic
Ceftaroline	600 mg IV q12h	CrCl 31–50: 400 mg q12h CrCl 15–30: 300 mg q12h CrCl <15 and HD: 200 mg q12h[a]	Fifth-generation cephalosporin
Dalbavancin	1500 mg IV ×1 or 1000 mg IV ×1 then 500 mg IV ×1 one week later	CrCl <30: 1125 mg IV ×1 or 750 mg IV ×1 then 375 mg IV ×1 one week later HD: N/A	Lipoglycopeptides Bactericidal activity
Oritavancin	1200 mg IV ×1	N/A	May falsely elevate: • aPTT for up to 5 days • ACT for up to 24 h • PT/INR for up to 12 h

Telavancin	10 mg/kg IV q24h	CrCl 30–50: 7.5 mg/kg IV q24h CrCl 10–29: 10 mg/kg IV q48h CrCl <10 and HD: not studied	Adverse effects include taste disturbance, nausea, vomiting, and renal dysfunction
Clindamycin	600 mg IV q8h or 300–450 mg PO QID	N/A	Use if clindamycin resistance <10–15% Bacteriostatic activity
Trimethoprim-sulfamethoxazole	One to two DS tablets PO BID	CrCl 15–30: 50% dose CrCl <15: avoid use	Reserve for mild infection Bactericidal activity
Doxycycline	100 mg PO bid	N/A	Reserve for mild infection Tetracycline; bacteriostatic
Minocycline	200 mg PO ×1 then 100 mg PO BID	N/A	"
Nonpurulent SSTI: *Streptococcus*			
Penicillin	2–4 mu IV q4–6h	CrCl >10 and uremia: 2–4 mu ×1 then 50% dose q4–6h CrCl <10 and HD: 2–4 mu ×1 then 50% dose q8h[a]	Bactericidal activity
Clindamycin	600–900 mg IV q8h	N/A	Bacteriostatic activity
Nafcillin	1–2 g IV q4–6h	N/A	Bactericidal activity

Continued

Table 11.6 Antimicrobial Therapy for SSTIs—cont'd

	STANDARD DOSING	RENAL DOSING	COMMENTS
Oxacillin	1–2 g IV q4–6h	N/A	Bactericidal activity
Cefazolin	1 g IV q8h	CrCl 11–34: 50% dose q12h CrCl ≤10 and HD: 50% dose q24h[a]	Cross-sensitivity with PCN allergy Bactericidal activity

Notes:
- Duration of therapy
  - 5 days for uncomplicated infection
  - Up to 14 days for severe infection, slow response to therapy, or immunosuppression
- Parenteral antimicrobial recommended if:
  - Extensive soft tissue infection
  - Signs of systemic toxicity
  - Rapid progression of infection
  - Persistence of symptoms despite 48 h of oral antimicrobial
  - Immunocompromise
  - Proximity of soft tissue infection to an indwelling medical device

ACT, Activated whole blood clotting time; aPTT, activated partial thromboplastin time; bid, Twice daily; BW, Body weight; CrCl, Creatinine clearance; DS, double strength; HD, Hemodialysis; INR, International normalized ratio; IV, intravenously; MIC, Minimum inhibitory concentration; MSSA, Methicillin-susceptible Staphylococcus aureus; mu, Million units; N/A, Not applicable; PCN, Penicillin; PO, Orally; PT, prothrombin time; qid, Four times daily
[a]Give post HD on HD days.
[b]Consult pharmacist for dosing
Data from Stevens DL, Bisno AL, Chambers HF, et al. Infectious Diseases Society of America. Practice guidelines for the diagnosis and management of skin and soft tissue infections: 2014 update by the Infectious Diseases Society of America. Clin Infect Dis. 2014;59(2):e10-52.

Table 11.7 Antimicrobial Therapy for Necrotizing Infections

PATHOGEN	ANTIMICROBIAL OF CHOICE	STANDARD DOSING (IV)	RENAL DOSING/COMMENTS
Polymicrobial			
Aerobic/anaerobic gram-positive and gram-negatives	Vancomycin plus	See Table 11.1 for dosing	Imipenem-cilastatin
	Piperacillin-tazobactam	3.375 g q6–8h	CrCl 60–8g: 500 mg q6h or 750 mg q8h
	Imipenem-cilastatin	1 g q6–8h	CrCl 30–59: 500 mg q6–8h
	Meropenem[a]	1 g q8h	CrCl 15–29 and HD: 500 mg q12h[b]
	Ertapenem[a]	1 g q24h	CrCl <15 without HD: avoid use
	Cefotaxime/metronidazole	2 g q6h/500 mg q6h	Cefotaxime
	or cefotaxime/clindamycin	2 g q6h/600–900 mg q8h	CrCl <20: 50% dose[b]
			Piperacillin-tazobactam
			CrCl 20–40: 2.25 g q6h
			CrCl <20: 2.25 g q8h
			HD: 2.25 g q12h[b]
Monomicrobial			
Streptococcus	Penicillin	2–4 mu q4–6h	Penicillin
	plus		CrCl >10 and uremia: 2–4 mu ×1 then 50% dose q4–6h
	Clindamycin	600–900 mg q8h	CrCl <10 and HD: 2–4 mu ×1 then 50% dose q8h[b]

Continued

Table 11.7 Antimicrobial Therapy for Necrotizing Infections—cont'd

PATHOGEN	ANTIMICROBIAL OF CHOICE	STANDARD DOSING (IV)	RENAL DOSING/COMMENTS
Staphylococcus aureus	Nafcillin	1–2 g q4h	—
	Oxacillin	1–2 g q4h	
	Cefazolin	1 g q8h[c]	
	Vancomycin	See Table 11.1 for dosing	
	Clindamycin	600–900 mg q8h	
Clostridium species, non–C. difficile clostridia	Penicillin plus	2–4 mu q4–6h	Penicillin: see above
	Clindamycin	600–900 mg q8h	
Aeromonas hydrophilia	Doxycycline plus	100 mg q12h	—
	Ciprofloxacin or	400 mg q12h[c]	
	Ceftriaxone	1–2 g q24h	
Vibrio vulnificus	Doxycycline plus	100 mg q12h	Cefotaxime: see above
	Ceftriaxone	1 g q24h	Ceftazidime
	Cefotaxime or	2 g q8h	CrCl 31–50: 1 g q12h
	Ceftazidime	1 g q8h	CrCl 16–30: 1 g q24h
			CrCl 6–15: 500 mg q24h
			CrCl <5: 500 mg q48h
			HD: 1 g ×1 then 500 mg q24h[b]

Notes:

- Alternative antimicrobial for severe penicillin allergy
  - Polymicrobial: clindamycin or metronidazole plus aminoglycoside or fluoroquinolone
  - *Streptococcus* or *Staphylococcus aureus*: vancomycin, linezolid, quinupristin/dalfopristin, or daptomycin
  - *Clostridium* species: clindamycin alone

CrCl, Creatinine clearance; *HD*, Hemodialysis; *IV*, Intravenously; *mu*, Million units

[a] See Table 11.2 for renal dosing

[b] Give post HD on HD days

[c] See Table 11.4 for renal dosing

Adapted from Stevens DL, Bisno AL, Chambers HF, et al. Infectious Diseases Society of America. Practice guidelines for the diagnosis and management of skin and soft tissue infections: 2014 update by the Infectious Diseases Society of America. *Clin Infect Dis.* 2014;59(2):e10–e52.

ANTIMICROBIAL PROPHYLAXIS IN SURGERY[7]

- Definitions:
  - Primary prophylaxis: prevention of an initial infection (focus of this section)
  - Secondary prophylaxis: prevention of recurrence of a previous infection
  - Eradication: elimination of a colonized organism to prevent an infection
- Administration time of preoperative dose: within 60 min before surgical incision
- Antimicrobial selection and dosing (Tables 11.8 and 11.9)
- Duration of prophylaxis: less than 24 h

BACTERIAL MENINGITIS[8]

- Definitions:
  - Community-acquired meningitis: an infection unrelated to a neurosurgical procedure, neurotrauma, or hospitalization.
  - Health care-acquired meningitis: an infection related to invasive procedures, cranial trauma, traumatic brain injury, and hematogenous spread with hospital-acquired bacteremia.
- Management:
  - Algorithm (Fig. 11.3)
  - Empiric antibiotic therapy (Table 11.10)
  - Pathogen and susceptibility specific antibiotic therapy (Table 11.11)
  - Antibiotic dosing (Table 11.12)

Table 11.8 Antibiotic Therapy for Surgical Prophylaxis

TYPE OF PROCEDURE	RECOMMENDED ANTIBIOTIC	ALTERNATIVE ANTIBIOTIC FOR β-LACTAM ALLERGY
Neurosurgery	Cefazolin	Clindamycin or vancomycin
Head and Neck		
Clean with placement of prosthesis (excludes tympanostomy tubes)	Cefazolin or cefuroxime	Clindamycin
Clean-contaminated procedures except for tonsillectomy and functional endoscopic sinus procedures	[Cefazolin + metronidazole], [cefuroxime + metronidazole], or ampicillin-sulbactam	Clindamycin
Cardiac	Cefazolin or cefuroxime	Clindamycin or vancomycin
Thoracic	Cefazolin or ampicillin-sulbactam	Clindamycin or vancomycin
Gastroduodenal	Cefazolin	[Clindamycin or vancomycin] + [AG or aztreonam or FQ]
Biliary tract (open procedure and high-risk laparoscopic procedure)	Cefazolin, cefoxitin, cefotetan, ceftriaxone, or ampicillin-sulbactam	[Clindamycin or vancomycin] + [AG or Aztreonam or FQ] or [metronidazole] + [AG or FQ]
Appendectomy for uncomplicated appendicitis	Cefoxitin, cefotetan, or [cefazolin + metronidazole]	[Clindamycin] + [AG or aztreonam or FQ] or [metronidazole] + [AG or FQ]

Continued

Table 11.8 Antibiotic Therapy for Surgical Prophylaxis—cont'd

TYPE OF PROCEDURE	RECOMMENDED ANTIBIOTIC	ALTERNATIVE ANTIBIOTIC FOR β-LACTAM ALLERGY
Small Intestine		
Nonobstructed	Cefazolin	[Clindamycin] + [AG or aztreonam or FQ]
Obstructed	[Cefazolin + metronidazole], cefoxitin, or cefotetan	[Metronidazole] + [AG or FQ]
Hernia repair	Cefazolin	Clindamycin or vancomycin
Colorectal	[Cefazolin + metronidazole], cefoxitin, cefotetan, ampicillin-sulbactam, [ceftriaxone + metronidazole], or ertapenem	[Clindamycin] + [AG or aztreonam or FQ] or [metronidazole] + [AG or FQ]
Orthopedic		
Clean operations involving hand, knee, or foot without implantation of foreign materials	None	None
All others	Cefazolin	Clindamycin or vancomycin
Cesarean delivery	Cefazolin	[Clindamycin + AG]
Hysterectomy (vaginal or abdominal)	Cefazolin, cefotetan, cefoxitin, or ampicillin-sulbactam	[Clindamycin or vancomycin] + [AG or aztreonam or FQ] or [metronidazole] + [AG or FQ]

Procedure	Recommended Agent	Alternative Agent
Urologic		
Lower tract instrumentation with risk factors for infection (includes transrectal prostate biopsy)	FQ, TMP-SMX, or cefazolin	AG ± clindamycin
Clean without entry into urinary tract	Cefazolin ± a single dose AG	Clindamycin or vancomycin
Involving implanted prosthesis	[Cefazolin] ± [AG or aztreonam] or ampicillin-sulbactam	[Clindamycin] ± [AG or aztreonam] or [vancomycin] ± [AG or aztreonam]
Clean with entry into urinary tract	Cefazolin ± a single dose AG	FQ or [AG ± clindamycin]
Clean-contaminated	[Cefazolin + metronidazole] or cefoxitin	FQ or [AG] + [metronidazole or clindamycin]
Vascular	Cefazolin	Clindamycin or vancomycin
Heart, lung, heart-lung transplantation	Cefazolin	Clindamycin or vancomycin
Liver transplantation	Piperacillin-tazobactam or [cefotaxime + ampicillin]	[Clindamycin or vancomycin] + [AG or aztreonam or FQ]
Pancreas and pancreas-kidney transplantation	Cefazolin or fluconazole (if high risk of fungal infection)	[Clindamycin or vancomycin] + [AG or aztreonam or FQ]
Plastic surgery	Cefazolin or ampicillin-sulbactam	Clindamycin or vancomycin

AG, Aminoglycoside; FQ, Fluoroquinolone; TMP-SMX, Trimethoprim-sulfamethoxazole
Adapted from Bratzler DW, Dellinger EP, Olsen KM, et al. Clinical practice guidelines for antimicrobial prophylaxis in surgery. Am J Health Syst Pharm. 2013;70(3):195–283.

Table 11.9 Antibiotic Dosing for Surgical Prophylaxis

ANTIBIOTIC	STANDARD DOSE (IV)	INTRAOPERA-TIVE REDOSING INTERVAL (H)	COMMENTS
Ampicillin	2 g	2	—
Ampicillin/ Sulbactam	3 g	2	Covers *Acinetobacter*
Aztreonam	2 g	4	Alternative for β-lactam allergy
Cefazolin	2 g 3 g if ≥ 120 kg	4	First line for many procedures
Cefuroxime	1.5 g	4	—
Cefotaxime	1 g	3	—
Cefoxitin	2 g	2	Some anaerobe activity
Cefotetan	2 g	6	Some anaerobe activity
Ceftriaxone	2 g	N/A	Hepatic clearance
Ciprofloxacin	400 mg	N/A	*Pseudomonas* coverage
Clindamycin	900 mg	6	—
Ertapenem	1 g	N/A	Cross-sensitivity with β-lactam allergy
Fluconazole	400 mg	N/A	—
Gentamicin	5 mg/kg	N/A	Consult pharmacist for dosing
Levofloxacin	500 mg	N/A	*Pseudomonas* coverage
Metronidazole	500 mg	N/A	—
Moxifloxacin	400 mg	N/A	No *Pseudomonas* coverage; has some anaerobe coverage

Table 11.9 Antibiotic Dosing for Surgical Prophylaxis—cont'd

ANTIBIOTIC	STANDARD DOSE (IV)	INTRAOPERATIVE REDOSING INTERVAL (H)	COMMENTS
Piperacillin/ tazobactam	3.375 g	2	*Pseudomonas* coverage
Vancomycin	15 mg/kg Max 2 g	N/A	Consult pharmacist for dosing

Notes:
- Oral antibiotics for colorectal surgery prophylaxis: neomycin 1g plus erythromycin base 1 g or metronidazole 1 g (no redosing)
- Intraoperative redosing recommended if procedure lasts >2 half-lives of the antimicrobial or excessive bleeding
- Vancomycin and fluoroquinolones are administered over ≥60 min; infusion should be started 120 min before surgical incision

H, Hour; *IV*, Intravenous; *N/A*, Not applicable.
Adapted from Bratzler DW, Dellinger EP, Olsen KM, et al. Clinical practice guidelines for antimicrobial prophylaxis in surgery. *Am J Health Syst Pharm.* 2013;70(3):195–283.

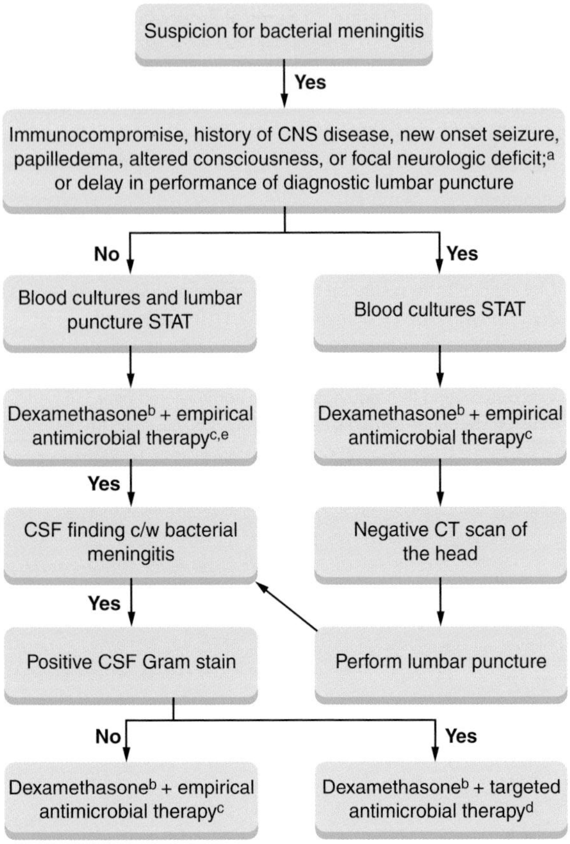

Figure 11.3 Management Algorithm for Suspected Bacterial Meningitis.
From Tunkel AR, Hartman BJ, Kaplan SL, Kaufman BA, et al. Clin Infect Dis. Practice guidelines for the management of bacterial meningitis. Clin Infect Dis. 2004;39:1267–1284.
[a]Recommended criteria for computed tomography (CT) prior to lumbar puncture. [b]Recommended for suspected or confirmed pneumococcal meningitis (see note in Table 11.11 for dosing). [c]See Table 11.10. [d]See Table 11.11. [e]Dexamethasone and antimicrobial therapy should be administered immediately after CSF is obtained. CSF: cerebrospinal fluid.

TABLE 11.10 Empiric Antibiotic Therapy for Bacterial Meningitis

PREDISPOSING FACTOR	COMMON PATHOGENS	EMPIRIC ANTIBIOTIC
Community Acquired		
18–50 years	*N. meningitidis* *S. pneumoniae*	Vancomycin + ceftriaxone or cefotaxime
>50 years	*N. meningitidis* *S. pneumoniae* *Listeria monocytogenes* Aerobic GNB	Vancomycin + ceftriaxone or cefotaxime + ampicillin
Health Care Acquired		
Basilar skull fracture	*S. pneumoniae* *H. influenzae* Group A β-hemolytic streptococci	Vancomycin + ceftriaxone or cefotaxime
Penetrating trauma	*S. aureus* CoNS Aerobic GNB (including PSA)	Vancomycin + cefepime or ceftazidime or meropenem
Post-neurosurgery	Aerobic GNB (including PSA) *S. aureus* CoNS	"
CSF shunt	CoNS *S. aureus* Aerobic GNB (including PSA) *Propionibacterium acnes*	"

Notes:
- Alternative for β-lactam allergy
  - Mild reaction to a cephalosporin: meropenem + vancomycin
  - Severe reaction to a penicillin and/or cephalosporin: moxifloxacin + vancomycin

CoNS, Coagulase-negative staphylococci; *GNB*, Gram-negative bacilli; *H. influenzae, Haemophilus influenzae; N. meningitidis, Neisseria meningitidis; PSA, Pseudomonas aeruginosa; S. aureus: Staphylococcus aureus; S. pneumoniae: Streptococcus pneumoniae*
Adapted from Tunkel AR, Hartman BJ, Kaplan SL, et al. Practice guidelines for the management of bacterial meningitis. *Clin Infect Dis.* 2004;39:1267–1284.

Table 11.11 Pathogen and Susceptibility Specific Antibiotic Therapy for Bacterial Meningitis

PATHOGEN	RECOMMENDED ANTIBIOTIC	ALTERNATIVE ANTIBIOTIC
Streptococcus pneumoniae		
Penicillin MIC (μg/mL)		
<0.1	Penicillin G or ampicillin	Ceftriaxone, cefotaxime, or chloramphenicol
0.1–1	Ceftriaxone or cefotaxime	Cefepime, meropenem
≥2	Vancomycin + ceftriaxone or cefotaxime[a]	Moxifloxacin
Cefotaxime or ceftriaxone MIC ≥1 μg/mL	Vancomycin + ceftriaxone or cefotaxime[a]	Moxifloxacin
Neisseria meningitidis		
Penicillin MIC (μg/mL)		
<0.1	Penicillin G or ampicillin	Ceftriaxone, cefotaxime, or chloramphenicol
0.1–1	Ceftriaxone or cefotaxime	Chloramphenicol, moxifloxacin, or meropenem
Listeria monocytogenes	Ampicillin or penicillin G[b]	TMP-SMX, meropenem
Streptococcus agalactiae	Ampicillin or penicillin G[b]	Ceftriaxone or cefotaxime
***Escherichia coli* and other enterobacteriaceae**	Ceftriaxone or cefotaxime	Aztreonam, moxifloxacin, meropenem, TMP-SMX, ampicillin
Pseudomonas aeruginosa	Cefepime[b] or ceftazidime[b]	Aztreonam,[b] ciprofloxacin,[b] meropenem[b]

Haemophilus Influenzae

| β-Lactamase negative | Ampicillin | Ceftriaxone, cefotaxime, cefepime, chloramphenicol, or moxifloxacin |
| β-Lactamase positive | Ceftriaxone or cefotaxime | Cefepime, chloramphenicol, or moxifloxacin |

Staphylococcus aureus

| Methicillin susceptible | Nafcillin or oxacillin | Vancomycin, meropenem |
| Methicillin resistant | Vancomycin[a] | TMP-SMX, Linezolid |

Staphylococcus epidermidis | Vancomycin[a] | Linezolid |

Enterococcus species

Ampicillin susceptible	Ampicillin + gentamicin	—
Ampicillin resistant	Vancomycin + gentamicin	—
Ampicillin/vancomycin resistant	Linezolid	—

Notes:

- Dexamethasone for suspected or confirmed pneumococcal meningitis: 0.15 mg/kg IV q6h ×2–4 days, with the first dose administered 10–20 min before, or at least at the time of the first dose of antibiotic
- Duration of therapy
  - *Streptococcus pneumoniae*, CoNS, *Staphylococcus aureus*, GNB, *Propionibacterium acnes*: 10–14 days
  - *Listeria monocytogenes*: at least 21 days

CoNS, Coagulase-negative staphylococci; *GNB*, Gram-negative bacilli; *MIC*, Minimum inhibitory concentration; *TMP-SMX*, Trimethoprim-sulfamethoxazole

[a]Consider adding rifampin

[b]Consider adding an aminoglycoside

Adapted from Tunkel AR, Hartman BJ, Kaplan SL, et al. Practice guidelines for the management of bacterial meningitis. *Clin Infect Dis.* 2004;39:1267–1284.

Table 11.12 Antibiotic Dosing for Bacterial Meningitis

ANTIBIOTIC	STANDARD DOSING (IV)	RENAL DOSING
Amikacin Standard doses: 250–750 mg (round to nearest 50 mg)	5 mg/kg q8h[a]	CrCl 20–60: 5 mg/kg q12–24h based on level CrCl <20 and HD: 5 mg/kg load then based on level[b]
Ampicillin 125 mg, 250 mg, 500 mg, 1 g, 2 g	2 g q4h	CrCl 10–50: 2 g q6h CrCl <10 and HD: 2 g q12h[b]
Aztreonam (Azactam) 1 g, 2 g	2 g q6–8h	CrCl 10–30: 1 g q6–8h CrCl <10: 500 mg q6–8h HD: 2 g LD, then 500 mg q6–8h[b]
Cefepime (Maxipime) 1 g, 2 g	2 g q8h	CrCl 30–60: 2 g q12h CrCl <30: 2 g q24h HD: 1 g q24h[b]
Cefotaxime (Claforan) 1 g, 2 g	2 g q4–6h	CrCl <20: 50% dose q4–6h HD: 2 g q24h[b]
Ceftazidime (Fortaz) 500 mg, 1 g, 2 g	2 g q8h	CrCl 31–50: 2 g q12h CrCl 16–30: 2 g q24h CrCl ≤15 and HD: 1 g q24h[b]

Drug	Dose	Renal adjustment
Ceftriaxone (Rocephin) 1 g, 2 g	2 g q12h	—
Chloramphenicol (Chloromycetin) 1 g	1–1.5 g q6h	Mild–severe impairment: use with caution
Ciprofloxacin (Cipro) 200 mg, 400 mg	400 mg q8–12h	CrCl 5–29 and HD: 400 mg q24h[b]
Gentamicin Standard doses: 60–120 mg (round to nearest 10 mg)	1.67 mg/kg q8h[a]	CrCl 20–60: 1.67 mg/kg q12–24h based on level CrCl <20 and HD: 1.67 mg/kg load, then based on level[b]
Linezolid (Zyvox) 600 mg	600 mg q12h[b]	Mild–severe impairment: use with caution
Meropenem (Merrem) 500 mg, 1 g	2 g q8h	CrCl 26–50: 2 g q12h CrCl 10–25: 1 g q12h CrCl <10: 1 g q24h HD: 500 mg q24h[b]
Moxifloxacin (Avelox) 400 mg	400 mg q24h	—
Nafcillin 1 g, 2 g	2 g q4h	—

Continued

Table 11.12 Antibiotic Dosing for Bacterial Meningitis—cont'd

ANTIBIOTIC	STANDARD DOSING (IV)	RENAL DOSING
Oxacillin (Bactocill) 1 g, 2 g	2 g q4h	—
Penicillin G (Pfizerpen) Standard doses: 1 mu, 2 mu, 3 mu, 4 mu	4 mu q4h	CrCl >10 and uremia: 50% dose CrCl <10: 4 mu ×1 then 50% dose q8h[b]
Rifampin (Rifadin) 600 mg	600 mg q24h	—
Tobramycin Standard doses: 60–120 mg (round to nearest 10 mg)	1.67 mg/kg q8h[a]	CrCl 20–60: 1.67 mg/kg q12–24h based on level CrCl <20 and HD: 1.67 mg/kg load, then based on level[b]
TMP-SMX (Bactrim) SMX 80 mg/TMP 16 mg/mL	5 mg/kg q6–12h	CrCl 10–30: 5 mg/kg q12h CrCl <10 and HD: 5 mg/kg q24h[b]
Vancomycin (Vancocin) Standardized doses: 0.5-2g (round to nearest 250mg)	15 mg/kg q8–12h[a]	CrCl 15–50: 750–1500 mg q24h CrCl <15: 750–1500 mg based on level HD: 500–1000 mg based on level[b]

CrCl, Creatinine clearance; *HD,* Hemodialysis; *IV,* Intravenously; *mu,* Million units; *TMP-SMX,* Trimethoprim-sulfamethoxazole
[a]Consult pharmacist for dosing
[b]Give post HD on HD days
Adapted from Tunkel AR, Hartman BJ, Kaplan SL, et al. Practice guidelines for the management of bacterial meningitis. *Clin Infect Dis.* 2004;39:1267–1284.

References

1. Kalil AC, Metersky ML, Klompas M, et al. Management of adults with hospital-acquired and ventilator-associated pneumonia: 2016 clinical practice guidelines by the Infectious Diseases Society of America and the American Thoracic Society. *Clin Infect Dis.* 2016;63(5):e61–e111.

2. Mandell LA, Wunderink RG, Anzueto A, et al.; Infectious Diseases Society of America; American Thoracic Society. Infectious Diseases Society of America/American Thoracic Society consensus guidelines on the management of community-acquired pneumonia in adults. *Clin Infect Dis.* 2007;44(S2):S27–S72.

3. Uyeki TM, Bernstein HH, Bradley JS, et al. Clinical practice guidelines by the Infectious Diseases Society of America: 2018 update on diagnosis, treatment, chemoprophylaxis, and institutional outbreak management of seasonal influenza. *Clin Infect Dis.* 2018;68(6):e1–e47.

4. Mermel LA, Allon M, Bouza E, et al. Clinical practice guidelines for the diagnosis and management of intravascular catheter-related infection: 2009 update by the Infectious Diseases Society of America. *Clin Infect Dis.* 2009;49:1–45.

5. Hooton TM, Bradley SF, Cardenas DD, et al. Diagnosis, prevention, and treatment of catheter-associated urinary tract infection in adults: 2009 international clinical practice guidelines from the Infectious Diseases Society of America. *Clin Infect Dis.* 2010;50(5):625–663.

6. Stevens DL, Bisno AL, Chambers HF, et al.; Infectious Diseases Society of America. Practice guidelines for the diagnosis and management of skin and soft tissue infections: 2014 update by the Infectious Diseases Society of America. *Clin Infect Dis.* 2014;59(2):e10–e52.

7. Bratzler DW, Dellinger EP, Olsen KM, et al. Clinical practice guidelines for antimicrobial prophylaxis in surgery. *Am J Health Syst Pharm.* 2013;70(3):195–283.

8. Tunkel AR, Hartman BJ, Kaplan SL, et al. Practice guidelines for the management of bacterial meningitis. *Clin Infect Dis.* 2004;39:1267–1284.

12

Sepsis and Septic Shock

This chapter will review the recommendations from the 2016 Surviving Sepsis Campaign by Society of Critical Care Medicine (SCCM) and European Society of Intensive Care Medicine (ESICM).

DEFINITIONS

- Sepsis: life-threatening organ dysfunction caused by a dysregulated inflammatory response to an infection.
- Septic shock: a severe form of sepsis characterized by circulatory, cellular, and metabolic dysfunction.

Organ Dysfunction Can Be Identified As A Change In The Sepsis-Related Organ Failure Assessment (SOFA) Score Of 2 Points Or Higher

- Quick-SOFA(Q-SOFA):
  - A predictive tool that calculates the risk of death from sepsis.
  - Three components, each of which are allocated one point:
    - Respiratory rate ≥22 per minute
    - Altered mentation
    - Systolic blood pressure ≤100 mm Hg
- A score ≥2 is associated with poor outcomes due to sepsis.

MANAGEMENT OF SEPSIS AND SEPTIC SHOCK[1]

Volume Resuscitation

Intravascular hypovolemia is typical and may be severe in sepsis. Rapid, large volume infusion is the cornerstone of initial resuscitation to achieve tissue perfusion.

Crystalloids (Table 12.1)

- 30 mL/kg within the first 3 h (each 1000 mL over 30 min), unless pulmonary edema
- Normal saline has a risk of hyperchloremic acidosis

Colloids

- Albumin 5% 250–500 mL over 30–60 min. Form: 5% (250 mL, 500 mL), 25% (50 mL, 100 mL)
- No difference in mortality when albumin compared with crystalloids
- Synthetic colloids (e.g., hydroxyethyl starch) are not recommended due to coagulopathy and risk of acute kidney injury

Vasopressors

- Use intravenous vasopressors if patients remain hypotensive despite adequate fluid resuscitation or patients develop cardiogenic pulmonary edema (Table 12.2)

Corticosteroids (3–7 days)

- For patients with septic shock refractory to adequate fluid resuscitation and vasopressor administration.
  - Hydrocortisone:
    - A pharmacologic form of cortisol
    - Most commonly used glucocorticoid in large randomized trials
    - Dose: 50 mg intravenous (IV) q6h.
  - The adrenocorticotropic hormone (ACTH) stimulation test has failed to consistently identify patients with septic shock who benefit from glucocorticoid use.

Table 12.1 Comparison of Crystalloids

SOLUTIONS	Na (mEq/L)	K (mEq/L)	Cl (mEq/L)	BUFFERS (mEq/L)	Ca (mEq/L)	Mg (mEq/L)	pH	OSMOLALITY (mOsm/L)
0.9% NaCl	154	—	154	—	—	—	5.7	308
Lactated Ringer	130	4	109	Lactate 28	2.7	—	6.5	274
PlasmaLyte, Normosol	140	5	98	Acetate 27 Gluconate 23	—	3	7.4	294

Na, Sodium; *K*, Potassium; *Cl*, Chloride; *Ca*, Calcium; *Mg*, Magnesium.

Table 12.2 Vasopressors

DRUG	RECEPTORS CLINICAL EFFECTS	POTENCY	STANDARD DOSING (IV)	COMMENTS
Norepinephrine (Levophed)	Alpha-1 Beta-1 Beta-2	+++ ++ ++	Start at 5 mcg/min Titrate by 2 mcg/min q1min to MAP 65 Maximum: 50 mcg/min	First-line If inadequate, add epinephrine or vasopressin
Epinephrine (Adrenalin)	Alpha-1 Beta-1 Beta-2 SVR	++ +++ ++ ++	Start at 5 mcg/min Titrate by 2.5 mcg/min q1omin to MAP 65 Maximum: 30 mcg/min	Useful for anaphylactic shock
Vasopressin (Pitressin)	V1, V2 SVR	N/A ++	0.03 units/min Do not titrate Range: 0.01–0.04 units/min Maximum: 0.04 units/min	Add to norepinephrine to improve MAP or decrease norepinephrine requirements
Dobutamine (Dobutrex)	Alpha-1 Beta-1 Beta-2 CO	+/– +++ ++ +	5 mcg/kg/min Do not titrate Range: 5–40 mcg/kg/min Maximum: 40 mcg/kg/min	First-choice inotrope May cause hypotension

Continued

Table 12.2 Vasopressors—cont'd

DRUG	RECEPTORS CLINICAL EFFECTS	POTENCY	STANDARD DOSING (IV)	COMMENTS
Dopamine	<5 mcg/kg/min		Start at 5 mcg/kg/min	Alternative to norepineph-
	Beta-1	+	Titrate by 5 mcg/kg/min q10min to MAP	rine if bradycardia and
	Dopamine	+ +	65	low risk of tachyarrhyth-
	CO	+	Maximum: 40 mcg/kg/min	mias
	5–10 mcg/kg/min			
	Alpha-1	+		
	Beta-1	+ +		
	Dopamine	+ +		
	SVR	+		
	CO	+		
	10–20 mcg/kg/min			
	Alpha-1	+ +		
	Beta-1	+ +		
	Dopamine	+ +		
	SVR	+ +		
Phenylephrine (Neosynephrin)	Alpha-1	+ + +	Start at 50 mcg/min	Consider for patients in
	SVR	+ +	Titrate by 10 mcg/min q1min to MAP 65	whom norepinephrine is CI
			Maximum: 180 mcg/min	due to arrhythmias or who
				have failed other agents

Legend	
Receptor	**Cardiovascular Effect**
Alpha-1	Vasoconstriction, inotropy
Beta-1	Inotropy, chronotropy
Beta-2	Vasodilation, bronchodilation, inotropy
Dopamine	Vasodilation, vasoconstriction
V1	Vasoconstriction
V2	Water reabsorption

CI, Contraindicated; *CO,* Cardiac output; *IV,* Intravenously; *MAP,* Mean arterial pressure; *N/A,* Not applicable; *SVR,* systemic vascular resistance
Drugs without brand names are denoted by generic name only

- Hydrocortisone 50 mg IV q6h and fludrocortisone 50 mcg NG every morning decreased 90-day all-cause mortality in septic shock.

Antimicrobials (7–10 days)

Recommend starting empiric broad spectrum IV antimicrobials (gram-negative and -positive organisms and, if suspected, fungi and viruses) within 1 h of presentation. For septic shock, recommend at least two antimicrobials from two different classes (i plus ii or iii; Table 12.3). Once pathogen identified and susceptibility data return, deescalate antibiotics.

Methicillin-Resistant *Staphylococcus aureus* (MRSA)

- Vancomycin
- If refractory or contraindication to vancomycin, daptomycin (nonpulmonary MRSA), linezolid, or ceftaroline

Pseudomonas (if *Pseudomonas* is a likely pathogen)

- β-Lactam/β-lactamase inhibitor (piperacillin-tazobactam, ticarbillin-clavulanate)
- Cephalosporin (ceftazidime, cefepime)
- Carbapenem (imipenem, meropenem)
- Fluoroquinolone (ciprofloxacin)
- Aminoglycoside (amikacin, gentamicin, tobramycin)
- Monobactam (aztreonam)

Non-*Pseudomonas* (if *Pseudomonas* is an unlikely pathogen)

- Cephalosporin (ceftriaxone, cefotaxime)

Venous Thromboembolism (VTE) Prophylaxis (Table 12.4)

- Sepsis increases risk for VTE
- Mechanical VTE prophylaxis recommended if pharmacologic agent contraindicated

Stress Ulcer Prophylaxis

Recommended in patients with sepsis or septic shock who have risk factors for gastrointestinal bleeding such as mechanical

Table 12.3 IV Antimicrobials

ANTIBIOTIC FORMS	STANDARD DOSING (IV)	RENAL DOSING	COMMENTS
Amikacin Standardized doses: 250–750 mg (round to nearest 50 mg)	CD: 5–7.5 mg/kg q8h ODD: 15–20 mg/kg q24h	CrCl 20–60: CD: 5–7.5 mg/kg q12–24h[a] ODD: 15–20 mg/kg q36–48h CrCl <20: CD: 5 mg/kg load then based on level ODD not recommended HD: 5 mg/kg[a,b] CRRT: 10 mg/kg load, then 7.5 mg/kg q24–48h[a]	Consult pharmacist for dosing Goal peak: 25–35 mcg/mL Goal trough: ≤8 mcg/mL Goal for ODD: refer to Hartford nomogram[c] Use ideal or adjusted BW for obese ADR: nephrotoxicity and ototoxicity
Aztreonam (Azactam) 1 g, 2 g	1–2 g q8h	CrCl 10–30: 1 g q8h CrCl <10: 500 mg q8h HD: 1–2 g LD, then 500 mg q12h[b] CRRT: 1 g q8h or 2 g q12h	Possible cross-sensitivity between aztreonam and ceftazidime (<5%); avoid aztreonam if history of life-threatening reaction or anaphylaxis to ceftazidime
Cefepime (Maxipime) 1 g, 2 g	2 g q8h	CrCl 30–60: 2 g q12h CrCl <30: 2 g q24h HD: 1 g q24h[b] CRRT: 1 g q8h or 2 g q12h	Risk of seizures in renal insufficiency

Continued

Table 12.3 IV Antimicrobials—cont'd

ANTIBIOTIC FORMS	STANDARD DOSING (IV)	RENAL DOSING	COMMENTS
Ceftazidime (Fortaz) 500 mg, 1 g, 2 g	2 g q8h	CrCl 31–50: 2 g q12h CrCl 16–30: 2 g q24h CrCl ≤15 & HD: 1 g q24h[b] CRRT: 1 g q8h or 2 g q12h	Possible cross-sensitivity between aztreonam and ceftazidime (<5%); avoid aztreonam if history of life-threatening reaction or anaphylaxis to ceftazidime
Cefotaxime (Claforan) 1 g, 2 g	2 g q6–8h	CrCl <20: Decrease dose by 50% HD: 1–2 g q24h[b] CRRT: 1–2 g q8h	10% cross-sensitivity with PCN allergy
Ceftaroline (Teflaro) 400 mg, 600 mg	600 mg q12h	CrCl 31–50: 400 mg q12h CrCl 15–30: 300 mg q12h CrCl <15: 200 mg q12h HD: 200 mg q12h[b] CRRT: 200 mg q12h	"
Ceftriaxone (Rocephin) 1 g, 2 g	1–2 g q24h[b]	No change	"

Drug	Standard dose	Renal/other adjustment	Notes
Ciprofloxacin (Cipro) 200 mg, 400 mg	400 mg q8h	CrCl 5–29 and HD: 400 mg q24h CRRT: 400 mg q12–24h	CI: myasthenia gravis, children due to musculoskeletal toxicity ADR: tendonitis/tendon rupture, QT prolongation, peripheral neuropathy, CNS effects, photosensitivity, hepatotoxicity, crystalluria
Daptomycin (Cubicin) 500 mg	6 mg/kg q24h Complicated bacteremia: 8–10 mg/kg q24h	CrCl <30 and HD: 6 mg/kg q48h[b] CRRT: 8 mg/kg q48h	Possible myopathy

Gentamicin Standardized doses: 60–120 mg (round to nearest 10 mg)	CD: 1–2.5 mg/kg q8–12h
	ODD: 5–7 mg/kg q24h
		CrCl 20–60:
		  CD: 1–2.5 mg/kg q12–24h[a]
		  ODD: 5–7 mg/kg q36–48h
		CrCl <20:
		  CD: 1–2.5 mg/kg LD, then based on level
		  ODD not recommended
		HD: 1.5–2 mg/kg[a,b]
		CRRT: 1.5–2 mg/kg q24–48h[a]
			Consult pharmacist for dosing
			Goal peak: 6–8 mcg/mL
			Goal trough: ≤1–2 mcg/mL
			Goal for ODD: refer to Hartford nomogram[c]
			Use ideal or adjusted BW for obese
			ADR: nephrotoxicity and ototoxicity

Continued

Table 12.3 IV Antimicrobials—cont'd

ANTIBIOTIC FORMS	STANDARD DOSING (IV)	RENAL DOSING	COMMENTS
Imipenem (Primaxin) 250 mg, 500 mg	500 mg q6h Maximum: 1 g q6h	CrCl 10–50: 500 mg q8–12h CrCl <10 and HD: 250–500 mg q12h[b] CRRT: 500 mg q6–8h	Cross-sensitivity with PCN allergy Consider decreasing dose in patients <70 kg to prevent seizures
Linezolid (Zyvox) 600 mg	600 mg q12h[b]	No change	DDI: DC SSRI 2 weeks before linezolid to reduce risk of serotonin syndrome ± toxicity
Meropenem (Merrem) 500 mg, 1 g	1–2 g q8h Extended infusion (off-label): 0.5–2 g over 3 h q8h	CrCl 26–50: 1–2 g q12h CrCl 10–25: 500 mg–1 g q12h CrCl <10: 500 mg–1 g q24h HD: 500 mg q24h[b] CRRT: 500 mg–1 g q8h	Cross-sensitivity with PCN allergy Consider reserving for risk of ESBL-producing pathogens
Piperacillin-tazobactam (Zosyn) 2.25 g, 3.375 g, 4.5 g	Non-PSA: 3.375 g q6h PSA: 4.5 g q6h	Non-PSA: CrCl 20–40: 2.25 g q6h CrCl <20: 2.25 g q8h HD: 2.25 g q12h[b] PSA: CrCl 20–40: 3.375 g q6h CrCl <20: 2.25 g q6h HD: 2.25 g q8h[b]	Off-label extended infusion: 3.375–4.5 g ×1 over 30 min, followed 4 h later by 4 h infusion q8h

Ticarbillin 3 g-clavulanate 0.1 g (Timentin) 3.1 g	<60 kg: 200–300 mg ticarcillin/kg/day in divided doses q4–6h ≥60 kg: 3.1 g q4–6h Maximum: 18 g daily	CrCl 30–60: 2 g of ticarcillin q4h CrCl 10–30: 2 g of ticarcillin q8h CrCl <10 and HD: 2 g of ticarcillin q12h[b] CRRT: 3.1 g q6h	Not available in U.S.
Tobramycin	Same as gentamicin		
Vancomycin (Vancocin) Standardized doses: 0.5–2 g (round to nearest 250 mg)	15–20 mg/kg q8–12h Consider 25–30 mg/kg LD Maximum: 2 g/dose	CrCl 15–50: 750–1500 mg q24h[a] CrCl <15: 750–1500 mg[a,b] HD: 500–1000 mg[a,b] CRRT: 15–25 mg/kg LD, then 1000 mg q24–48h[a]	Consult pharmacist for dosing Goal trough: 15–20 mcg/mL Use actual BW for obese

ADR, Adverse drug reaction; BW, Body weight; CD, Conventional dosing; CI, Contraindicated; CrCl, Creatinine clearance; CRRT, Continuous renal replacement therapy; DC, Discontinue; DDI, Drug-drug interaction; ESBL, Extended-spectrum beta-lactamase; HD, Intermittent hemodialysis; IV, Intravenously; LD, Loading dose; ODD, Once daily dosing; PCN, Penicillin; PSA, Pseudomonas; SSRI, Selective serotonin-reuptake inhibitor

[a]Based on level
[b]Give post HD on HD days
[c]Fig. 10.1

Drugs without brand names are denoted by generic name only

Table 12.4 Pharmacologic VTE Prophylaxis

ANTICOAGULANT	STANDARD DOSE (SUBCUTANEOUS)	DOSE ADJUSTMENT
Low-Molecular-Weight Heparin (Preferred)		
Enoxaparin (Lovenox) 30 mg, 40 mg	40 mg q24h	CrCl <30 mL/min: 30 mg q24h Dialysis: avoid use
Dalteparin (Fragmin) 2500, 5000, 7500, 10,000, 12,500, 15,000, 18,000 units	5000 units q24h	Severe renal impairment: use with caution
Tinzaparin (Innohep) 2500, 3500, 4500 anti-Xa units Canada; not available in U.S.	4500 anti-Xa units q24h	CrCl <30 mL/min: use with caution
Nadroparin (Fraxiparine) 9500 anti-Xa units/Ml Canada; not available in U.S.	≤70 kg: 3800 anti-Xa units q24h >70 kg: 5700 anti-Xa units q24h	CrCl <30 mL/min: reduce dose by 25–33%
Unfractionated Heparin		
Heparin 5000 units	5000 units q8–12h	Frequency based on risk of thrombosis and bleeding
Factor Xa Inhibitor (If History of HIT)		
Fondaparinux (Arixtra) 2.5 mg	2.5 mg q24h	CrCl 30–50: 1.5 mg q24h CrCl <30 mL/min: contraindicated

CrCl, Creatinine clearance; *HIT,* Heparin-induced thrombocytopenia; *VTE,* Venous thromboembolism

ventilation >48 h, coagulopathy, preexisting liver disease, need for renal replacement therapy, and higher organ failure scores.

- Proton pump inhibitors: preferred (Table 12.5)
- Histamine-2-receptor antagonists (H2 blocker): second line (see Table 12.5)

Table 12.5 Stress Ulcer Prophylaxis

DRUG	STANDARD DOSE	DOSE ADJUSTMENT
Proton Pump Inhibitors (Preferred)		
Esomeprazole (Nexium) 20 mg, 40 mg	20 mg IV/PO/ NG daily	Oral: severe renal impairment: not recommended Oral and IV: severe hepatic impairment (Child-Pugh class C): maximum 20 mg daily
Dexlansoprazole (Dexilant) 30 mg, 60 mg	30 mg PO daily	N/A
Lansoprazole (Prevacid) 15 mg, 30 mg	30 mg PO/NG daily	Severe hepatic impairment (Child-Pugh class C): 15 mg once daily
Omeprazole (Prilosec) 10 mg, 20 mg, 40 mg	20 mg PO/NG daily	Mild to severe hepatic impairment (Child-Pugh class A, B, or C): 20 mg daily
Pantoprazole (Protonix) 20 mg, 40 mg	40 mg IV/PO/ NG daily	none
Rabeprazole (Aciphex) 5 mg, 10 mg, 20 mg	20 mg PO daily	Severe hepatic impairment (Child-Pugh class C): avoid use
Histamine-2-Receptor Antagonists (Second Line)		
Cimetidine (Tagamet) 200 mg, 300 mg, 400 mg, 800 mg, 300 mg/5 mL	300 mg PO/NG QID	Severe renal impairment: 300 mg q12h Hepatic impairment: use with caution Many drug-drug interaction

Continued

Table 12.5 Stress Ulcer Prophylaxis—cont'd

DRUG	STANDARD DOSE	DOSE ADJUSTMENT
Famotidine (Pepcid) 10 mg, 20 mg, 40 mg, 40 mg/5 mL	20 mg PO/IV/ NG BID	CrCl <50 mL/min: 20 mg daily or 10 mg BID
Nizatidine (Axid) 15 mg/mL, 75 mg, 150 mg, 300 mg	150 mg PO BID or 300 mg PO Qhs	CrCl 10–50 mL/min: 150 mg q24–48h CrCl <10 mL/min: 150 mg q48–72h HD: 150 mg q48–72h Peritoneal dialysis: 150 mg q48–72h

BID, Twice daily; *CrCl*, Creatinine clearance; *HD*, Hemodialysis; *IV*, Intravenously; *N/A*, Not applicable; *NG*, Nasogastric; *PO*, Orally; *Qhs*, Every night; *QID*, Four times daily

References

1. Rhodes A, Evans LE, Alhazzani W, et al. Surviving sepsis campaign: international guidelines for management of sepsis and septic shock: 2016. *Crit Care Med.* 2017;45(3):486–552.
2. Annane D, Renault A, Brun-Buisson C, et al. Hydrocortisone plus Fludrocortisone for Adults with Septic Shock. *N Engl J Med.* 2018;378:809–818.

Neurocritical Care

13

Acute Ischemic Stroke (AIS)

This chapter will review the drug therapy to treat ischemic stroke according to the 2018 American Heart Association/American Stroke Association Guidelines on Acute Ischemic Stroke.

DEFINITIONS

Stroke

An acute brain disorder of vascular origin with neurological dysfunction lasting >24 h.

Transient ischemic attack (TIA)

An acute ischemia with focal neurological dysfunction lasting <24 h.

CLASSIFICATION OF STROKE TYPES (FIG. 13.1)

NATIONAL INSTITUTES OF HEALTH STROKE SCALE (TABLE 13.1)

A quantitative assessment of stroke severity to help assess appropriateness of thrombolytic therapy.

MANAGEMENT

The Golden Hour for Acute Ischemic Stroke (AIS)

The time period following a stroke during which there is the highest probability that prompt medical treatment will be most effective to prevent death (Fig. 13.2)

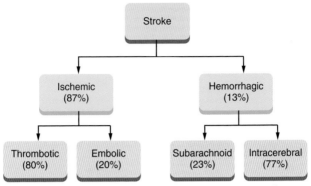

Figure 13.1 Classification of Stroke Types. *Data from Go AS, Mozaffarian D, Roger VL, et al. American Heart Association Statistics Committee and Stroke Statistics Subcommittee. Heart disease and stroke statistics–2013 update: a report from the American Heart Association. Circulation. 2013;127:e6–e245.*

Table 13.1 National Institutes of Health Stroke Scale (NIHSS)

CATEGORY	SCORE
1a. Level of Consciousness	0 = Alert
	1 = Drowsy
	2 = Stuporous
	3 = Coma
1b. Orientation questions[a]	0 = Answers both correctly
	1 = Answers one correctly
	2 = Incorrect
1c. Response to commands[a]	0 = Performs both correctly
	1 = Performs one correctly
	2 = Incorrect
2. Gaze	0 = Normal
	1 = Partial gaze palsy
	2 = Forced deviation
3. Visual Fields	0 = No visual loss
	1 = Partial hemianopia
	2 = Complete hemianopia
	3 = Bilateral hemianopia
4. Facial Paresis	0 = Normal
	1 = Minor
	2 = Partial
	3 = Complete

Table 13.1 National Institutes of Health Stroke Scale
(NIHSS)—cont'd

CATEGORY	SCORE
5a. Motor Arm—Left **5b. Motor Arm—Right**	0 = No drift 1 = Drift 2 = Can't resist gravity 3 = No effort against gravity 4 = No movement
6a. Motor Leg—Left **6b. Motor Leg—Right**	0 = No drift 1 = Drift 2 = Can't resist gravity 3 = No effort against gravity 4 = No movement
7. Limb Ataxia	0 = No ataxia 1 = Present in one limb 2 = Present in two limbs
8. Sensory	0 = Normal 1 = Partial loss 2 = Severe loss
9. Language	0 = No aphasia 1 = Mild-mod aphasia 2 = Severe aphasia 3 = Mute
10. Dysarthria	0 = Normal articulation 1 = Mild to mod slurring of words 2 = Near to unintelligible or worse
11. Extinction and Inattention	0 = No neglect 1 = Partial neglect 2 = Complete neglect

[a]Adapted from Lyden P, Brott T, Tilley B, et al. Improved reliability of the NIH Stroke Scale using video training. NINDS TPA Stroke Study Group. *Stroke.* 1994;25:2220–2226.

Pharmacologic Treatment for AIS

If symptom onset <4.5 h:

- Thrombolytic therapy: criteria for use (Table 13.2)
- Blood pressure management if alteplase eligible (Table 13.3)
- Alteplase dosing (Table 13.4)

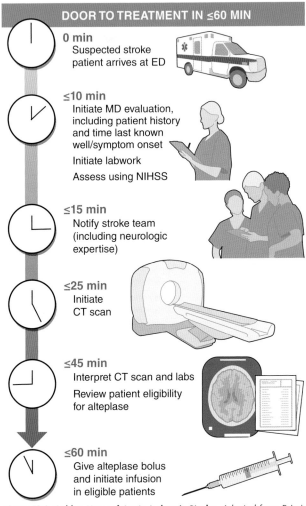

DOOR TO TREATMENT IN ≤60 MIN

0 min
Suspected stroke patient arrives at ED

≤10 min
Initiate MD evaluation, including patient history and time last known well/symptom onset

Initiate labwork

Assess using NIHSS

≤15 min
Notify stroke team (including neurologic expertise)

≤25 min
Initiate CT scan

≤45 min
Interpret CT scan and labs

Review patient eligibility for alteplase

≤60 min
Give alteplase bolus and initiate infusion in eligible patients

Figure 13.2 Golden Hour of Acute Ischemic Stroke. *Adapted from Brissie MA. The War Against Warfarin: Evaluating Current Treatment Guidelines for Patients Who Have Had an Acute Ischemic Stroke and Are Taking Warfarin. J Em Nursing (38)2:2012;188–92. CT,* Computed tomography; *ED,* Emergency department; *MD,* Medical doctor; *NIHSS,* National Institutes of Health Stroke Scale.

Table 13.2 Criteria for Alteplase use in Acute Ischemic Stroke (AIS)

Inclusion Criteria

- Age ≥18 yr
- Clinical diagnosis of ischemic stroke causing measurable neurological deficit
- Time of symptom onset well established to be <4.5 h before treatment would begin

Exclusion Criteria

- Current intracranial hemorrhage
- Subarachnoid hemorrhage
- Active internal bleeding
- Intracranial or intraspinal surgery or serious head trauma within the previous 3 months
- Presence of intracranial conditions that may increase the bleeding risk (e.g., some neoplasms, arteriovenous malformation, or aneurysms)
- Bleeding diathesis
- Current severe uncontrolled hypertension (e.g., SBP ≥185 mm Hg or DBP ≥110 mm Hg) despite treatment
- Treatment dose of LMWH within the previous 24 h
- Coagulopathy:
  - Platelets <100,000/mm³
  - INR >1.7, aPTT >40 s, or PT > 15 s
- Arterial puncture at noncompressible site within the previous 7 days
- Abnormal blood glucose (<50 mg/dL or >400 mg/dL)

Relative Exclusion Criteria

- Recent major surgery or procedure within the previous 14 days
- Cerebrovascular disease
- Recent intracranial hemorrhage
- Gastrointestinal or genitourinary bleeding within the previous 21 days
- Recent trauma
- Hypertension: SBP >175 mm Hg or DBP >110 mm Hg
- Possible left heart thrombus (e.g., mitral stenosis with atrial fibrillation)
- Acute pericarditis
- Subacute bacterial endocarditis
- Hemostatic defects
- Pregnancy
- Hemorrhagic ophthalmic conditions
- Septic thrombophlebitis or occluded AV cannula at infected site
- Advanced age >77 years

Continued

Table 13.2 Criteria for Alteplase use in Acute Ischemic Stroke (AIS)—cont'd

Relative Exclusion Criteria

- Concurrent anticoagulants
  - Use of heparin in past 48 h and elevated aPTT
  - Use of warfarin and INR >1.7 or PT ≥15 s
  - Use of direct thrombin inhibitors (e.g., dabigatran) or direct factor Xa inhibitors (e.g., rivaroxaban) within the previous 48 h
- Major surgery or serious trauma excluding head trauma within the previous 14 days
- MI, stroke, serious head trauma, or any intracranial surgery within the previous 3 months
- Structural GI malignancy
- Concurrent glycoprotein IIb/IIIa inhibitors
- Additional exclusion for treatment between 3 and 4.5 h: NIHSS >25
- Rapidly improving or minor stroke symptoms

Start Alteplase Immediately if Criteria Met

aPTT, Activated partial thromboplastin time; *AV,* Atrioventricular; *DBP,* Diastolic blood pressure; *GI,* Gastrointestinal; *INR,* International normalized ratio; *LMWH,* Low-molecular-weight heparin; *MI,* Myocardial infarction; *NIHSS,* National Institutes of Health Stroke Scale; *PT,* Prothrombin time; *SBP,* Systolic blood pressure.
Adapted from Powers WJ, Rabinstein AA, Ackerson T, et al., on behalf of the American Heart Association Stroke Council. 2018 Guidelines for the early management of patients with acute ischemic stroke: a guideline for healthcare professionals from the American Heart Association/American Stroke Association. *Stroke.* 2018;49:e46–e99.

Table 13.3 Blood Pressure Management in Patients With AIS Who Are Eligible for Alteplase

BLOOD PRESSURE (mm Hg)	DRUG AND DOSING REGIMEN
SBP >185 or DBP >110	• Labetalol 10–20 mg IV over 1–2 min, may repeat once after 10 min • Nicardipine 5 mg/h, titrate up by 2.5 mg/h q5–15min, max 15 mg/h • Clevidipine 1–2 mg/h, titrate by doubling dose q2–5min, max 21 mg/h • Other agents (e.g., hydralazine, enalaprilat) may be considered
SBP >180–230 or DBP >105–120	• Labetalol 10 mg IV over 1–2 min, then 2–8 mg/min • Nicardipine 5 mg/h, titrate up by 2.5 mg/h q5–15min, max 15 mg/h • Clevidipine 1–2 mg/h, titrate by doubling dose q2–5min, max 21 mg/h

Table 13.3 Blood Pressure Management in Patients With AIS Who Are Eligible for Alteplase—cont'd

BLOOD PRESSURE (mm Hg)	DRUG AND DOSING REGIMEN
DBP >140	• Nitroprusside 0.2–0.5 mcg/kg/min, titrate by 0.5 mcg/kg/min q5min, max 10 mcg/kg/min

Notes:
- Monitor BP q15min during and after IV alteplase ×2 h, then q30min ×6 h, then q1h until 24 h after IV alteplase treatment
- Maintain BP ≤180/105 mm Hg during and after alteplase

AIS, Acute ischemic stroke; *BP,* Blood pressure; *DBP,* Diastolic blood pressure; *IV,* Intravenously; *SBP,* Systolic blood pressure
Adapted from Powers WJ, Rabinstein AA, Ackerson T, et al., on behalf of the American Heart Association Stroke Council. 2018 Guidelines for the early management of patients with acute ischemic stroke: a guideline for healthcare professionals from the American Heart Association/ American Stroke Association. *Stroke.* 2018;49:e46–e99.

Table 13.4 IV Administration of Alteplase for AIS

Dosing weight: patient's actual weight (kg)
Total dose: 0.9 mg/kg (max 90 mg)
Bolus dose 1: 0.09 mg/kg (max 9 mg) IV push over 1 min then
Infusion dose 2: 0.81 mg/kg (max 81 mg) IV over 60 min

Notes:
- No anticoagulant/antithrombotic agents within 24 h of alteplase administration
- No invasive procedures within 24 h of alteplase administration
- Follow-up noncontrast head CT 24 h after alteplase if plan for anticoagulants or antiplatelet agents

AIS, Acute ischemic stroke; *CT,* Computerized tomography; *IV,* Intravenously; *max,* Maximum
Adapted from Powers WJ, Rabinstein AA, Ackerson T, et al., on behalf of the American Heart Association Stroke Covuncil. 2018 Guidelines for the early management of patients with acute ischemic stroke: a guideline for healthcare professionals from the American Heart Association/ American Stroke Association. *Stroke.* 2018;49:e46–e99.

If symptom onset ≥4.5 h:
- Low-risk TIA or moderate to major ischemic stroke: aspirin 162–325 mg daily
- High-risk TIA or minor ischemic stroke: aspirin 81–325 mg ×1 then 81 mg daily plus clopidogrel 300 mg ×1 then 75 mg daily ×21 days, followed by clopidogrel 75 mg daily alone[4]

Other recommendations:
- If TIA or ischemic stroke with atrial fibrillation, antico-agulate if indicated (see Chapter 4)
- Start or continue high-intensity statin therapy
- Start prophylaxis for deep venous thrombosis and pulmonary embolism (Table 12.4)

References

1. Go AS, Mozaffarian D, Roger VL, et al. American Heart Association Statistics Committee and Stroke Statistics Subcommittee. Heart disease and stroke statistics—2013 update: a report from the American Heart Association. *Circulation.* 2013;127:e6–e245.
2. Lyden P, Brott T, Tilley B, et al. Improved reliability of the NIH Stroke Scale using video training. NINDS TPA Stroke Study Group. *Stroke.* 1994;25:2220–2226.
3. Powers WJ, Rabinstein AA, Ackerson T, et al. On behalf of the American Heart Association Stroke Council. 2018 Guidelines for the early management of patients with acute ischemic stroke: a guideline for healthcare professionals from the American Heart Association/American Stroke Association. *Stroke.* 2018;49:e46–e99.
4. Wang YJ, Wang YL, Zhao X, et al., for the CHANCE Investigators. Clopidogrel with aspirin in acute minor stroke or transient ischemic attack. *N Engl J Med.* 2013;369:11–19.

14

Other Neurocritical Care

This chapter will review the pharmacotherapy for management of myasthenia crisis, Guillain-Barre syndrome, and antithrombotic-induced intracranial hemorrhage according to expert opinion.

MYASTHENIA CRISIS[1]

Definitions

Myasthenia Gravis (MG)

Autoimmune disease targeting acetylcholine receptors on the postsynaptic side of neuromuscular junctions.

Myasthenia Crisis

Worsening of MG with respiratory failure.

Precipitating Factors

- Respiratory infection
- Emotional stress
- Physiological stress (e.g., trauma, surgery)
- Tapering of immunosuppressants
- Drugs: aminoglycosides, fluoroquinolones, macrolides, tetracyclines, neuromuscular blocking agents, magnesium, β-blockers, verapamil, procainamide, quinidine

Management (Table 14.1)

Table 14.1 Common Therapies for MG

DRUG	STANDARD DOSING	ONSET OF BENEFIT	TIME TO PEAK BENEFIT	COMMENTS
Rapid Immunotherapies				
Plasma exchange	—	1–7 days	1–3 weeks	Directly removes acetylcholine receptor antibodies More effective and works faster than IVIG (2016 international consensus statement by the Myasthenia Gravis Foundation of America)
Intravenous immunoglobulin (IVIG)	0.4 g/kg IV daily × 5 days or 1 g/kg IV daily ×1–2 days	1–2 weeks	1–3 weeks	Clinical trials show equivalence to plasma exchange
Symptomatic Therapy				
Pyridostigmine	PO: 60–120 mg q6h IV/IM: 2–4 mg q6h (off-label)	10–15 min	2 h	Acetylcholinesterase inhibitor Hold during myasthenia crisis requiring mechanical ventilation to reduce airway secretions; restart at a lower dose after response to plasma exchange or IVIG

Table 14.1 Common Therapies for MG—cont'd

DRUG	STANDARD DOSING	ONSET OF BENEFIT	TIME TO PEAK BENEFIT	COMMENTS
Chronic Immunotherapies (PO)				
Prednisone	Initial: 20 mg daily Target: 1 mg/kg/ day Max: 100 mg/day	2–3 weeks	5–6 months	For patients who remain symptomatic on pyridostigmine Most commonly used initial immunosuppressant due to rapid onset
Azathioprine	1–3 mg/kg/ day	6–12 months	1–2 yr	First-line steroid-sparing agent Avoid in active liver disease and lymphopenia Monotherapy or in conjunction with glucocorticoids and/or pyridostigmine
Mycophenolate	0.5–1.5 g BID	6–12 months	1–2 yr	Alternative to azathioprine Avoid in lymphopenia Monotherapy or in conjunction with glucocorticoids and/or pyridostigmine
Cyclosporine	2.5 mg/kg BID	~6 months	~12 months	Second-line Monotherapy or in conjunction with glucocorticoids and/or pyridostigmine
Tacrolimus	3–5 mg daily			
Surgery				
Thymectomy	—	1–10 yr	1–10 yr	

BID, Twice daily; *IM*, Intramuscularly; *IV*, Intravenously; *max*, Maximum; *MG*, Myasthenia gravis; *PO*, Orally
Data from Sanders DB, Wolfe GI, Benatar M, et al. International consensus guidance for management of myasthenia gravis. *Neurology.* 2016;87(4):419–425.

GUILLAIN-BARRE SYNDROME[2]

Definition

Subacute inflammatory demyelinating polyneuropathy, often preceded by a respiratory infection, characterized by ascending paresthesias and ascending symmetric limb weakness, progression to respiratory failure, and autonomic instability.

Causes

Campylobacter jejuni, Epstein-Barr virus, varicella-zoster, mycoplasma pneumoniae infections

Management

- Supportive care
- Plasmapheresis: equivalent to intravenous immunoglobulin (IVIG)
- IVIG 0.4 g/kg/day × 5 days (European Federation of Neurological Societies)
- Glucocorticoids are not effective

ANTITHROMBOTIC-INDUCED INTRACRANIAL HEMORRHAGE[3]

Introduction

The use of antithrombotic agents, including anticoagulants, antiplatelets, and thrombolytics increases the risk of intracranial hemorrhage.

Management

Rapid reversal with the following therapeutic agents (Table 14.2) may help to control hematoma expansion and improve outcomes.

Table 14.2 Reversal of Antithrombotic Agents in Intracranial Hemorrhage

ANTITHROMBOTIC AGENTS	REVERSAL AGENTS*
Vitamin K antagonists Warfarin (Coumadin)	If INR ≥1.4: vitamin K 10 mg IV + 3 or 4 factor PCC IV If PCC unavailable, FFP 10–15 mL/kg IV

Direct factor Xa inhibitors
Apixaban (Eliquis)
Betrixaban (Bevyxxa)
Edoxaban (Lixiana)
Rivaroxaban (Xarelto)
	Activated charcoal 50 g within 2 h of ingestion
	Activated PCC (Feiba) or 4 factor PCC 50 units/kg IV
	Andexanet alfa (IV):
	  If apixaban or rivaroxaban >7 h: 400 mg bolus then 4 mg/min ×120 min
	  If edoxaban or rivaroxaban within 7 h or unknown time: 800 mg bolus then 8 mg/min ×120 min

Direct thrombin inhibitors Argatroban (Acova) Bivalirudin (Angiomax) Dabigatran (Pradaxa) Desirudin (Iprivask)	For dabigatran: activated charcoal 50 g within 2 h of ingestion + idarucizumab 2.5 g IV in 50 mL ×2 doses For other DTIs: activated PCC (Feiba) or 4 factor PCC 50 units/kg IV
Unfractionated heparin	Protamine 1 mg IV per 100 units of heparin in the previous 2–3 h Maximum protamine dose: 50 mg

LMWH
Enoxaparin (Lovenox)
Dalteparin (Fragmin)
	Enoxaparin:
	  Dosed within 8 h: protamine 1 mg IV per 1 mg of enoxaparin
	  Dosed within 8–12 h: protamine 0.5 mg IV per 1 mg of enoxaparin
	  Minimal use if dosed >12 h
	Dalteparin:
	  Dosed within 3–5 t ½: protamine 1 mg IV per 100 units of dalteparin
	  Maximum protamine dose: 50 mg
	  If protamine contraindicated: rFVIIa 90 mcg/kg IV

Pentasaccharides Fondaparinux (Aristra)	Activated PCC (Feiba) 20 units/kg IV or rFVIIa 90 mcg/kg IV

Continued

Table 14.2 Reversal of Antithrombotic Agents in Intracranial Hemorrhage—cont'd

ANTITHROMBOTIC AGENTS	REVERSAL AGENTS[a]

Thromblytic agents
Alteplase (Activase)
Reteplase (Retavase)
Tenecteplase (TNKase)
	Cryoprecipitate 10 units IV
	If cryoprecipitate contraindicated:
	  tranexamic acid 10–15 mg/kg IV over
	  20 min or aminocaproic acid 4–5 g IV

Antiplatelet agents Aspirin (Bayer Aspirin) Cangrelor (Kengreal) Clopidogrel (Plavix) Prasugrel (Effient) Ticagrelor (Brilinta)	Desmopressin; 0.4 mcg/kg IV ×1 If neurosurgical intervention: platelet transfusion

DTIs, Direct thrombin inhibitors; *FFP,* Fresh frozen plasma; *INR,* International normalized ratio; *IV,* Intravenously; *LMWH,* Low-molecular weight heparin; *PCC,* Prothrombin complex concentrates; *rFVIIa,* Recombinant factor VIIa; *t ½,* Half-life elimination
[a]See Table 24.10 for details
Adapted from Frontera JA, Lewin JJ 3rd, Rabinstein AA, et al. Guideline for reversal of antithrombotics in intracranial hemorrhage: a statement for healthcare professionals from the Neurocritical Care Society and Society of Critical Care Medicine. *Neurocrit Care.* 2016;24(1):6–46.

References

1. Sanders DB, Wolfe GI, Benatar M, et al. International consensus guidance for management of myasthenia gravis. *Neurology.* 2016;87(4):419–425.

2. Hughes RAC, Wijdicks EFM, Barohn R, et al. Practice parameter: immunotherapy for Guillain-Barre syndrome: report of the Quality Standards Subcommittee of the American Academy of Neurology. *Neurology.* 2003;61(6):736–740. Reaffirmed 2016.

3. Frontera JA, Lewin JJ 3rd, Rabinstein AA, et al. Guideline for reversal of antithrombotics in intracranial hemorrhage: a statement for healthcare professionals from the Neurocritical Care Society and Society of Critical Care Medicine. *Neurocrit Care.* 2016;24(1):6–46.

15

Status Epilepticus

This chapter will review recommendations from the 2012 Neurocritical Care Society and 2016 American Epilepsy Society Guidelines.

Definition

Status epilepticus is defined as 5 min of continuous seizures, or two seizures without regaining consciousness in between for more than 5 min.

Common Etiologies

See Table 15.1.

Management

- Treatment algorithm (Fig. 15.1)
- Pharmacotherapy (Table 15.2)

Table 15.1 Typical Etiologies of Status Epilepticus in the Intensive Care Unit

MOST COMMON	LESS COMMON
Drug Toxicity	**Ischemic**
• Amphetamines	• Stroke
• Cocaine	• Cardiac arrest
• Tricyclics	**Traumatic**
Drug Withdrawal	• Intracranial hemorrhage
• Barbiturates	• Intracranial hypertension
• Benzodiazepines	**Infectious**
• Ethanol	• Abscess
• Opiates	• Meningoencephalitis
Metabolic	• Septic emboli
• Hypoglycemia	**Hematologic**
• Hypoxia	• Disseminated intravascular coagulopathy
• Uremia	• Thrombotic thrombocytopenia purpura
• Liver failure	

Adapted from Brophy GM, Bell R, Claassen J, et al.; Neurocritical Care Society Status Epilepticus Guideline Writing Committee. Guidelines for the evaluation and management of status epilepticus. *Neurocrit Care.* 2012;17(1):3–23.

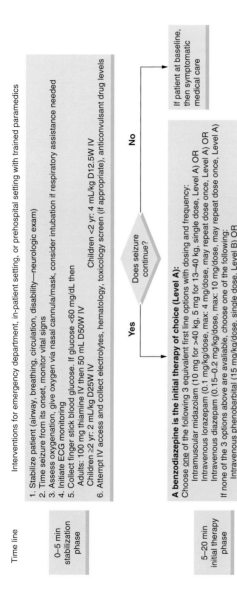

Time line

0–5 min stabilization phase

Interventions for emergency department, in-patient setting, or prehospital setting with trained paramedics

1. Stabilize patient (airway, breathing, circulation, disability—neurologic exam)
2. Time seizure from its onset, monitor vital signs
3. Assess oxygenation, give oxygen via nasal cannula/mask, consider intubation if respiratory assistance needed
4. Initiate ECG monitoring
5. Collect finger stick blood glucose. If glucose <60 mg/dL then
   Adults: 100 mg thiamine IV then 50 mL D50W IV
   Children ≥2 yr: 2 mL/kg D25W IV   Children <2 yr: 4 mL/kg D12.5W IV
6. Attempt IV access and collect electrolytes, hematology, toxicology screen (if appropriate), anticonvulsant drug levels

Does seizure continue?

Yes

No

If patient at baseline, then symptomatic medical care

5–20 min initial therapy phase

A benzodiazepine is the initial therapy of choice (Level A):
Choose one of the following 3 equivalent first line options with dosing and frequency:
Intramuscular midazolam (10 mg for >40 kg, 5 mg for 13–40 kg, single dose, Level A) OR
Intravenous lorazepam (0.1 mg/kg/dose, max: 4 mg/dose, may repeat dose once, Level A) OR
Intravenous diazepam (0.15–0.2 mg/kg/dose, max: 10 mg/dose, may repeat dose once, Level A)
If none of the 3 options above are available, choose one of the following;
Intravenous phenobarbital (15 mg/kg/dose, single dose, Level B) OR
Rectal diazepam (0.2–0.5 mg/kg, max: 20 mg/dose, single dose, Level B) OR
Intranasal midazolam (Level B), buccal midazolam (Level B)

Figure 15.1 Treatment Algorithm for Status Epilepticus by 2016 American Epilepsy Society Guidelines. *ECG,* Electrocardiography; *EEG,* Electroencephalography; *IV,* Intravenous *Level A,* Established as effective; *Level B,* Probably effective; *Level U,* Data inadequate or insufficient. *From Glauser T, Shinnar S, Gloss D, Arya R, Bainbridge J, Bare M, Bleck T, Dodson WE, Garrity L, Jagoda A, Lowenstein D, Pellock J, Riviello J, Sloan E, Treiman DM. Evidence-based guideline: treatment of convulsive status epilepticus in children and adults: report of the guideline committee of the American Epilepsy Society. Epilepsy Currents. 2016;16(1);48-61.*

Continued

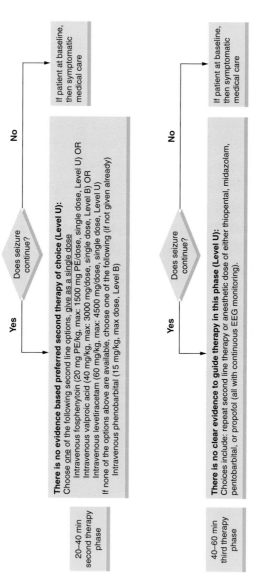

20–40 min second therapy phase

Yes

Does seizure continue?

No

There is no evidence based preferred second therapy of choice (Level U):
Choose one of the following second line options, give as a single dose
Intravenous fosphenytoin (20 mg PE/kg, max: 1500 mg PE/dose, single dose, Level U) OR
Intravenous valproic acid (40 mg/kg, max: 3000 mg/dose, single dose, Level B) OR
Intravenous levetiracetam (60 mg/kg, max: 4500 mg/dose, single dose, Level U)
If none of the options above are available, choose one of the following (if not given already)
Intravenous phenobarbital (15 mg/kg, max dose, Level B)

If patient at baseline, then symptomatic medical care

40–60 min third therapy phase

Yes

Does seizure continue?

No

There is no clear evidence to guide therapy in this phase (Level U):
Choices include: repeat second line therapy or anesthetic dose of either thiopental, midazolam, pentobarbital, or propofol (all with continuous EEG monitoring).

If patient at baseline, then symptomatic medical care

Figure 15.1 cont'd

Table 15.2 Drug Regimens for Generalized Status Epilepticus

DRUG	USUAL DOSE	PD/PK	METABOLISM	COMMENTS
First-Line Therapy (Emergency): Benzodiazepine				
Lorazepam	0.1 mg/kg IV (up to 4 mg/dose), MR in 5–10 min NTE: 2 mg/min	Onset: 10 min Duration: 6–8 h Half-life: 14 h	Hepatic	IV formulation contains propylene glycol ADR: sedation, hypotension, respiratory depression
Midazolam	0.2 mg/kg IM up to 10 mg/dose	Onset: 15 min Duration: up to 6 h Half-life: 3 h	Hepatic; active metabolite	Short duration with IV ADR: sedation, hypotension, respiratory depression
Diazepam	0.15 mg/kg IV up to 10 mg/dose, MR in 5 min NTE: 5 mg/min If IV not available, 0.2–0.5 mg/kg PR up to 20 mg/dose	Onset: IV: 1–3 min PR: 2–10 min Duration: 15–30 min Half-life: IV: parent 33–45 h; desmethyl-diazepam: 100 h PR: parent 45–46 h; desmethyl-diazepam: 71–99 h	Hepatic Active metabolites: N-desmethyl-diazepam, temazepam, and oxazepam	IV formulation contains propylene glycol Not recommended as first-line therapy due to short duration of seizure control ADR: sedation, hypotension, respiratory depression

Continued

Table 15.2 Drug Regimens for Generalized Status Epilepticus—cont'd

DRUG	USUAL DOSE	PD/PK	METABOLISM	COMMENTS
Second-Line Therapy (Urgent): Initiate After Benzodiazepine if Seizures Persist or if a Maintenance Needed				
Valproate	20–40 mg/kg IV, up to 3000 mg/dose	Time to peak: at the end of 1 h infusion Half-life: 9–19 h	Hepatic	Therapeutic level: 50–100 mcg/mL
Phenytoin	20 mg/kg IV, may give additional 5 mg/kg 10 min after LD NTE: 50 mg/min	Onset: 0.5–1 h Half-life: 7–42 h	Dose-dependent (Michaelis-Menten) PK	Enzyme inducer; several DDIs IV formulation contains propylene glycol and ethanol ADR: hypotension, arrhythmia, phlebitis, purple glove syndrome, hepatotoxicity Only compatible in saline
Fosphenytoin	20 PE mg/kg IV, may give additional 5 mg/kg 10 min after LD Max: 1500 mg PE/dose NTE: 150 mg/min May also give IM	Time to peak: 15 min Half-life: Fosphenytoin: 15 min Phenytoin: 12–29 h	Hepatic; fosphenytoin is rapidly converted to phenytoin via hydrolysis	Enzyme inducer; several DDIs ADR: hypotension, arrhythmia, hepatotoxicity

Drug	Dose	Pharmacokinetics	Metabolism	Comments
Phenobarbital	20 mg/kg IV, may give additional 5–10 mg/kg 10 min after LD NTE: 100 mg/min	Onset: 5 min Duration: >6 h Half-life: 53–118 h	Hepatic	IV formulation contains propylene glycol Enzyme inducer ADR: sedation, hypotension, respiratory depression
Levetiracetam	1–3 g or 60 mg/kg IV up to 4500 mg/dose NTE: 5 mg/kg/min	Time to peak: 1 h Half-life: 6–8 h	Enzymatic hydrolysis (24% of dose) Renal excretion (66% as unchanged and 27% as inactive metabolites)	ADR: sedation, paradoxical excitation, irritability Renally eliminated
Third-Line Therapy (Refractory): Initiate if Seizures Persist After First- and Second-Line Therapy				
Midazolam high-dose infusion	0.05–0.2 mg/kg/h	Onset: 3–5 min Half-life: 1.8–6.8 h (prolonged in renal failure, cirrhosis, CHF, obesity, and elderly)	Hepatic, active metabolite	Requires intubation before starting therapy ADR: sedation, hypotension, respiratory depression

Continued

Table 15.2 Drug Regimens for Generalized Status Epilepticus—cont'd

DRUG	USUAL DOSE	PD/PK	METABOLISM	COMMENTS
Pentobarbital	25 mg/kg LD followed by 0.5–5 mg/kg/h	Onset: 3–5 min Half-life: 15–50 h (dose dependent)	Hepatic	Requires intubation before starting therapy IV formulation contains propylene glycol Enzyme inducer; several DDIs ADR: sedation, hypotension, respiratory/cardiac depression, paralytic ileus, immunosuppression
Propofol	20–200 mcg/kg/min Titrate by 5 mcg/kg/min q5min	Onset: 9–51 s Half-life: Biphasic: Initial: 40 min Terminal: 4–7 h (after 10-day infusion, may be up to 1–3 days)	Hepatic	Requires intubation before starting therapy ADR: sedation, hypotension, respiratory depression, pancreatitis, cardiac failure, rhabdomyolysis, metabolic acidosis, propofol infusion syndrome Lipid formulation provides 1.1 kcal/mL

Valproate	20–40 mg/kg IV, may give additional 20 mg/kg 10 min after LD NTE: 5 mg/kg/min	Hepatic	Time to peak: at the end of a 1 h infusion Half-life: 9–19 h	For nonintubated Many DDIs, avoid in patients with a TBI ADR: hyperammonemia, thrombocytopenia, hepatotoxicity, pancreatitis
Lacosamide	200–400 mg IV NTE: 200 mg/15 min	Renal excretion (95%)	Time to peak: 1–4 h Half-life: 13 h	For nonintubated ADR: dizziness, bradyarrhythmia, PR prolongation, hypotension
Topiramate	200–400 mg PO/NG ×1 then 300–1600 mg/day PO/NG (divided two to four times daily)	Renal excretion (70% as unchanged drug)	Time to peak: 2 h Half-life: 19–23 h	For nonintubated ADR: metabolic acidosis No IV formulation available
Ketamine	0.5–5 mg/kg/h	Hepatic	Onset: 30 s Half-life: α: 10–15 min β: 2.5 h	ADR: excitation, hypertension, possible neurotoxicity, hallucinations

ADR, Adverse drug reaction; *CHF*, Congestive heart failure; *DDI*, Drug-drug interaction; *IM*, Intramuscularly; *IV*, Intravenously; *LD*, Loading dose; *MR*, May repeat; *NG*, Nasogastric; *NTE*, Not to exceed; *PD/PK*, Pharmacodynamics/pharmacokinetics; *PE*, Phenytoin equivalent; *PO*, Orally; *PR*, Per rectum; *TBI*, Traumatic brain injury

Adapted from Brophy GM, Bell R, Claassen J, et al.; Neurocritical Care Society Status Epilepticus Guideline Writing Committee. Guidelines for the evaluation and management of status epilepticus. *Neurocrit Care*. 2012;17(1):3–23; Glauser T, Shinnar S, Gloss D, et al. Evidence-based guideline: treatment of convulsive status epilepticus in children and adults: report of the guideline committee of the American Epilepsy Society. *Epilepsy Currents*. 2016;16(1):48–61.

References

1. Brophy GM, Bell R, Claassen J, et al.; Neurocritical Care Society Status Epilepticus Guideline Writing Committee. Guidelines for the evaluation and management of status epilepticus. *Neurocrit Care.* 2012;17(1):3–23.
2. Glauser T, Shinnar S, Gloss D, et al. Evidence-based guideline: treatment of convulsive status epilepticus in children and adults: report of the Guideline Committee of the American Epilepsy Society. *Epilepsy Currents.* 2016;16(1):48–61.

Pulmonary
Disorders

16

Asthma and Chronic Obstructive Pulmonary Disease (COPD) Exacerbation

This chapter will review the recommendations from the 2007 National Asthma Education and Prevention Program Guidelines and Global Initiative for Chronic Obstructive Lung Disease 2019.

ASTHMA EXACERBATION

Definition

An acute or subacute episode of worsening shortness of breath, cough, wheezing, and chest tightness, or a combination of these symptoms.

Mortality Risk Factors

- Previous severe exacerbation (e.g., intubation or intensive care unit admission for asthma).
- Two or more hospitalizations or three or more emergency department (ED) visits in the previous year.
- Hospitalization or ED visit for asthma in the past month.
- Use of more than two canisters of short-acting β-agonists per month.
- Difficulty perceiving asthma symptoms or severity of exacerbations.
- Social history that includes major psychosocial problems, illicit drug use, low socioeconomic status.
- Concomitant illnesses including cardiovascular diseases, psychiatric illness, or other chronic lung diseases.

Pharmacotherapy

See Table 16.1

CHRONIC OBSTRUCTIVE PULMONARY DISEASE (COPD) EXACERBATION

Definition

A change in the patient's baseline dyspnea, cough, or sputum production necessitating additional treatment.

Common Causes of Acute COPD Exacerbation

- Respiratory tract infection (most common).
  - Bacterial: *Streptococcus pneumoniae, Haemophilus influenzae, Moraxella catarrhalis.*
  - Viral: influenza, rhinovirus, parainfluenza, respiratory syncytial virus.
- Medication noncompliance.
- Temperature change.
- Air pollution.

Management

- Oxygen therapy.
- Mechanical ventilation: noninvasive or invasive.
- Pharmacologic Management.
  - Acute therapy (Table 16.2).
  - Maintenance therapy (Table 16.3).

Table 16.1 Drugs for Asthma Exacerbations

DRUG	DOSAGE	COMMENTS
Inhaled Short-Acting β2-Agonists (SABA): cornerstone in management of acute, severe asthma. MOA: stimulate β2 receptors causing relaxation of respiratory smooth muscle, leading to bronchodilation and a decrease in airway obstruction.		
Albuterol		
Nebulizer solution (2.5 mg/3 mL, 5 mg/mL)	2.5–5 mg q20min ×3, then 2.5–10 mg q1–4h PRN or 10–15 mg/h continuously	May mix with ipratropium nebulizer solution
MDI or dry powder inhaler (90 mcg/puff)	Four to eight puffs q20min up to 4h, then q1–4h PRN	Wait 15 s between actuations
Levalbuterol		
Nebulizer solution (1.25 mg/0.5 mL, 1.25 mg/3 mL)	1.25–2.5 mg q20min ×3, then 1.25–5 mg q1–4h PRN	Continuous nebulization not evaluated Levalbuterol one-half the mg dose of albuterol provides comparable efficacy and safety
MDI (45 mcg/puff)	See albuterol MDI dose	
Systemic β2-Agonists (Subcutaneous): if no response to inhaled therapy after a few hours.		
Epinephrine 1:1,000 (1 mg/mL)	0.3–0.5 mg q20min ×3	No proven advantage of systemic therapy over aerosol
Terbutaline (1 mg/mL)	0.25 mg q20min ×3	
Anticholinergics: given in combination with SABA MOA: bind to muscarinic receptors on respiratory smooth muscle, leading to reduction in bronchoconstriction		

Continued

Table 16.1 Drugs for Asthma Exacerbations—cont'd

DRUG	DOSAGE	COMMENTS
Ipratropium bromide Nebulizer solution (0.25 mg/mL) MDI (18 mcg/puff)	0.5 mg q20min ×3, then PRN Eight puffs q20min PRN up to 3 h	Not a first-line therapy; should be added to SABA for severe exacerbations May mix with albuterol nebulizer solution
Ipratropium with albuterol Nebulizer solution (0.5 mg/2.5 mg per vial) MDI (18 mcg/90 mcg per inhalation)	3 mL q20min ×3, then PRN Eight puffs q20min PRN up to 3 h	Adding ipratropium to albuterol has shown benefit in severe exacerbations, not in mild or moderate exacerbations
Systemic Corticosteroids: for moderate-severe exacerbations or for patients with inadequate response to SABA treatment. MOA: decrease airway obstruction by reducing inflammation and airway edema, increase the number of β2 receptors and their responsiveness to β-agonists, and suppress proinflammatory cytokines.		
Prednisone	40–80 mg/day in one to two divided doses until PEF 70% of predicted or personal best	Duration: 3–10 days (no tapering necessary)
Methylprednisolone		
Prednisolone		

Notes:

- Methylxanthines and mucolytics are not recommended in acute exacerbation due to increased side effect profiles and a lack of efficacy
- Antibiotics are not recommended in acute exacerbation except as needed for comorbid condition such as pneumonia or sinusitis
- May consider magnesium sulfate 2 g infused over 20 min for severe exacerbation refractory to initial therapy

MDI, Metered dose inhaler; *MOA,* Mechanism of action; *PEF,* Peak expiratory flow; *PRN,* As needed
Adapted from National Asthma Education and Prevention Program. *Expert Panel Report III: Guidelines for the Diagnosis and Management of Asthma.* Bethesda, MD. National Heart, Lung, and Blood Institute; 2007. (NIH publication no. 08-4051). www.nhlbi.nih.gov/guidelines/asthma/asthgdln.htm. (Accessed July 26, 2019).

Table 16.2 Pharmacologic Treatment in Acute COPD Exacerbation

DRUG	DOSAGE	COMMENTS
Inhaled Short-Acting β2-Agonists (SABA): initial bronchodilators for acute treatment of COPD exacerbation.		
Albuterol Nebulizer solution (2.5 mg/3 mL, 5 mg/mL) MDI or dry powder inhaler (90 mcg/inhalation)	2.5 mg nebulized q1–4h PRN One inhalation q1h ×2–3, then q2–4h PRN	Continue or start as soon as possible: inhaled long acting bronchodilators (β₂-agonists or anticholinergics or combination) ± inhaled corticosteroids (Table 16.3)
Levalbuterol Nebulizer solution (1.25 mg/0.5 mL, 1.25 mg/3 mL) MDI (45 mcg/inhalation)	1.25 mg nebulized q1–4h PRN See albuterol MDI dose	Levalbuterol one-half the mg dose of albuterol provides comparable efficacy and safety
Anticholinergics: given in Combination With SABA		
Ipratropium bromide Nebulizer solution (0.25 mg/mL) MDI (18 mcg/inhalation)	0.5 mg nebulized q6–8h Two inhalations q4–6h	Should not be used as first-line therapy; should be added to SABA for severe exacerbations May mix with albuterol nebulizer solution
Corticosteroids		
Prednisone, Prednisolone	40 mg PO daily	PO route preferred
Methylprednisolone	60–125 mg IV in one to four divided doses or 32 mg PO daily	PO prednisolone equally effective as IV Budesonide nebulization provides similar benefits to IV methylprednisolone Duration of therapy: 5–7 days
Budesonide (0.25 mg/2 mL; 0.5 mg/2 mL; 1 mg/2 mL)	2 mg nebulized q6h	

Continued

Table 16.2 Pharmacologic Treatment in Acute COPD Exacerbation—cont'd

DRUG	DOSAGE	COMMENTS
Antibiotics		
If risk factors for *pseudomonas*:		Antibiotics indicated if:
Levofloxacin	750 mg PO/IV daily	–Increase in dyspnea, sputum volume, and
Cefepime	2 g IV q8h	sputum purulence
Ceftazidime	2 g IV q8h	–Increase in sputum purulence and one of
Piperacillin-tazobactam	4.5 g IV q6h	the other two symptoms above
		–Require mechanical ventilation
If no risk factors for *pseudomonas*:		Duration of therapy: 5–7 days
Levofloxacin	500 mg PO/IV daily	Choose antibiotic based on local bacterial
Moxifloxacin	400 mg PO/IV daily	resistance pattern
Ceftriaxone	1–2 g IV daily	Deescalate or escalate based on final C/S
Cefotaxime	1–2 g IV q8h	

Notes:
- Belgian trial with Azithromycin during acute COPD exacerbations (BACE), phase 3 trial: azithromycin 500 mg daily ×3 days then 250 mg q2d ×90 days initiated at the time of hospitalization may decrease ICU and hospital stay
- Methylxanthines are not recommended in acute exacerbation due to increased side effect profiles and a lack of efficacy

COPD, Chronic obstructive pulmonary disease; *C/S*, Cultures and sensitivities; *ICU*, Intensive care unit; *IV*, Intravenously; *MDI*, Metered dose inhaler; *PO*, Orally; *PRN*, As needed
Data from Global Initiative for Chronic Obstructive Lung Disease (GOLD). *Global Strategy for the Diagnosis, Management and Prevention of Chronic Obstructive Pulmonary Disease;* 2019 Report. http://www.goldcopd.org. Accessed July 26, 2019.

Table 16.3 Pharmacologic Treatment in Stable COPD

DRUG	DOSAGE	COMMENTS
Inhaled Long-Acting β₂-Agonists (LABA): relax bronchial smooth muscle and antagonize bronchoconstriction		
Arfomoterol (Brovana) Nebulizer solution (15 mcg/2 mL)	15 mcg nebulized BID	Continue long-acting bronchodilators (β2-agonists or anticholinergics or combinations) with or without inhaled corticosteroids during exacerbation or start as soon as possible
Formoterol Foradil dry powder inhaler (12 mcg capsule) Perforomist nebulizer solution (20 mcg/2 mL)	12 mcg inhaled q2h 20 mcg nebulized BID	
Indacaterol (Arcapta Neohaler) Dry powder inhaler (75 mcg capsule)	1 capsule inhaled daily via approved inhalation device	LAMA may be superior to LABA regarding exacerbation prevention
Olodaterol (Striverdi Respimat) Aerosol solution (2.5 mcg/inhalation)	Two inhalations daily	
Salmeterol (Serevent Diskus) Aerosol powder (50 mcg/inhalation)	One inhalation BID	

Continued

Table 16.3 Pharmacologic Treatment in Stable COPD—cont'd

DRUG	DOSAGE	COMMENTS
Long-Acting Muscarinic Antagonists (LAMA): block bronchoconstriction in bronchial smooth muscle		
Aclidinium bromide (Tudorza Pressair) Aerosol Powder (400 mcg/inhalation)	One inhalation BID	LAMAs have a greater reduction on exacerbation rates compared with LABAs
Glycopyrronium bromide Seebri Neohaler (15.6 mcg capsule) Lonhala Magnair nebulizer solution (25 mcg/mL)	One capsule inhaled BID One vial nebulized BID	Decrease hospitalizations
Tiotropium Spiriva HandiHaler dry powder (18 mcg capsule) Spiriva Respimat soft-mist (2.5 mcg/inhalation)	One capsule inhaled daily Two inhalations daily	
Umeclidinium (Incruse Ellipta) Aerosol powder (62.5 mcg/inhalation)	One inhalation daily	
Combination Short-Acting β₂-Agonists + Muscarinic Antagonist (SABA/SAMA)		
Albuterol/ipratropium (Combivent Respimat®) 100 mcg/20 mcg per inhalation 2.5 mcg/0.5 mcg per 3 mL vial	One inhalation QID One vial nebulized q6h	SABA/SAMA combination superior to either drug alone

Combination Long-Acting β₂-Agonists + Muscarinic Antagonist (LABA/LAMA)

Formoterol/glycopyrronium (Bevespi Aerosphere)
4.8 mcg/9 mcg per inhalation
Two inhalations BID — LABA/LAMA combination increases FEV₁ and reduces symptoms and exacerbations compared to monotherapy

Indacaterol/glycopyrronium (Utibron Neohaler)
27.5 mcg/15.6 mcg per capsule
One inhalation BID

Vilanterol/umeclidinium (Anoro Ellipta)
Aerosol powder (25 mcg/62.5 mcg per inhalation)
One inhalation daily

Olodaterol/tiotropium (Stiolto Respimat)
Aerosol solution (2.5 mcg/2.5 mcg per inhalation)
Two inhalations daily

Combination of Long-Acting β₂-Agonists + Inhaled Corticosteroids (LABA/ICS)

Formoterol/budesonide (Symbicort)
MDI (4.5 mcg/160 mcg per inhalation)
Two inhalations BID — Consider adding ICS for patients with exacerbations despite long-acting bronchodilators

Formoterol/mometasone (Dulera)
5 mcg/100 mcg, 5 mcg/200 mcg per inhalation
Two inhalations BID — LABA/ICS recommended if blood eosinophil counts ≥300 cells/μL or history of asthma

Salmeterol/fluticasone (Advair Diskus)
Powder, 50 mcg/250 mcg per inhalation
One inhalation BID

Vilanterol/fluticasone furoate (Breo Ellipta)
25 mcg/100 mcg, 25 mcg/200 mcg per inhalation
One inhalation daily

Continued

Table 16.3 Pharmacologic treatment in stable COPD—cont'd

DRUG	DOSAGE	COMMENTS
Triple Combination (LABA/LAMA/ICS)		
Fluticasone/umeclidinium/vilanterol (Trelegy Ellipta) Aerosol powder (100 mcg/62.5 mcg/25 mcg per inhalation)	One inhalation daily	Improves lung function, symptoms, and health status and reduces exacerbations compared to LABA/ICS, LABA/LAMA, or LAMA
Methylxanthines: non-specific inhibitors of all phosphodiesterase enzyme subsets		
Theophylline Capsule extended release 24 h, oral Tablet extended release 12 h, oral Solution 80 mg/15 mL, oral	300–600 mg/day in divided doses, titrate to serum level 8–12 mcg/mL	Exerts a small bronchodilator effect in stable COPD Third-line agent in chronic COPD Dose-related toxicity such as ar-rhythmias, grand mal convulsions DDI with commonly used drugs such as digoxin, warfarin, etc.
Phosphodiesterase-4 Inhibitor		
Roflumilast	250 mcg daily ×4 weeks then 500 mcg daily	Consider in patients with FEV_1 <50% predicted and chronic bronchitis Avoid in hepatic impairment or history of moderate–severe depression

Antibiotics for Prevention of Exacerbations: for patients with frequent exacerbations despite maximal COPD therapy		
Azithromycin (preferred over Erythromycin due to better side effect and drug interaction profiles and broader spectrum of activity)	250–500 mg TIW or 250 mg daily	For former smokers, not currently smoking Reduce exacerbations over 1 year Macrolides are associated with increased bacterial resistance, QT prolongation, and hearing loss
Erythromycin	200–400 mg per day (formulation not specified) or 250 mg (stearate) BID	
Mucoregulators and Antioxidant Agents		
Acetylcysteine nebulization	Not routinely recommended for COPD	
Adjunct therapies supporting prevention and maintenance in COPD		
• Smoking cessation • Influenza and pneumococcal vaccinations • Proper inhaler technique		

BID, Twice daily; *COPD*, Chronic obstructive pulmonary disease; *DDI*, Drug-drug interaction; *FEV₁*, Forced expiratory volume in one second; *MDI*, Metered dose inhaler; *QID*, Four times daily; *TIW*, Three times weekly.

Data from Global Initiative for Chronic Obstructive Lung Disease (GOLD). *Global Strategy for the Diagnosis, Management and Prevention of Chronic Obstructive Pulmonary Disease*; 2019 Report. http://www.goldcopd.org. Accessed July 26, 2019.

References

1. National Asthma Education and Prevention Program. *Expert Panel Report III. Guidelines for the Diagnosis and Management of Asthma*. Bethesda, MD: National Heart, Lung, and Blood Institute; 2007. NIH publication no. 08-4051. www.nhlbi.nih.gov/guidelines/asthma/asthgdln.htm. Accessed July 26, 2019.
2. Global Initiative for Chronic Obstructive Lung Disease (GOLD). Global Strategy for the Diagnosis, Management and Prevention of Chronic Obstructive Pulmonary Disease; 2019 Report. http://www.goldcopd.org. Accessed July 26, 2019.

17

Pulmonary Arterial Hypertension (Group 1 Pulmonary Hypertension)

This chapter will review the pharmacotherapy for treatment of pulmonary arterial hypertension (PAH) according to the 2019 CHEST Guideline.

Definitions

- Pulmonary hypertension (PH) is characterized by mean pulmonary arterial pressure (mPAP) $\geq$20 mm Hg at rest and pulmonary vascular resistance three or more wood units measured by right heart catheterization. The World Health Organization (WHO) classifies PH into five groups based on etiologies (Table 17.1).
- PAH is Group 1 PH caused by idiopathic and heritable causes, drugs, connective tissue disease, congenital heart

Table 17.1 World Health Organization of Clinical Classification of PH

Group 1	PAH
Group 2	PH caused by left heart disease
Group 3	PH caused by lung disease and/or hypoxia
Group 4	Chronic thromboembolic PH
Group 5	Unclear multifactorial mechanisms

PAH, Pulmonary arterial hypertension; *PH*, Pulmonary hypertension
Adapted from Simonneau G, Robbins IM, Beghetti M, et al. Updated clinical classification of pulmonary hypertension. *J Am Coll Cardiol.* 2009;54:S43–S54.

Table 17.2 World Health Organization of Functional Class (WHO-FC)

CLASS	DEFINITION
I	No symptoms (dyspnea, fatigue, syncope, chest pain) with normal activities
II	Symptoms with strenuous normal daily activities; slight limitations in functional status/activity level
III	Symptoms with normal daily activities; severe limitation in functional status/activity level
IV	Symptoms at rest; unable to perform normal daily activities without symptoms

Adapted from Rubin LJ, American College of Chest Physicians. Diagnosis and management of pulmonary arterial hypertension: ACCP evidence-based clinical practice guidelines. *Chest.* 2004;126(1 suppl):7S–10S.

disease, human immunodeficiency virus, portopulmonary hypertension, schistosomiasis, pulmonary venoocclusive disease, or PH of the newborn.

Functional Class

See Table 17.2

Management of PAH

Supportive Therapy

- Oxygen: maintain SaO_2 ≥90% and PaO_2 ≥60 mm Hg.
- Diuretics: for the symptomatic management of right ventricular (RV) dysfunction and fluid overload.
- Digoxin: consider in atrial tachyarrhythmias.
- Anticoagulation: may consider in idiopathic PAH, heritable PAH, and PAH secondary to anorexigenic agent use (conflicting data).

Treatment Algorithm

See Fig. 17.1

Vasodilator Therapy With Calcium Channel Blockers if Demonstrates Acute Vasoreactivity.

- Diltiazem extended-release (ER) 240–720 mg daily.
- Amlodipine up to 20 mg daily.
- Nifedipine ER 120–240 mg daily.

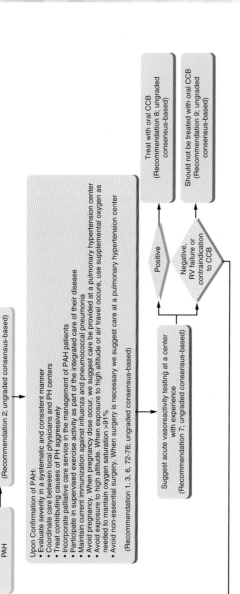

Patients with suspected PAH

→

Evaluate promptly at PH center
(Recommendation 2; ungraded consensus-based)

↓

Upon Confirmation of PAH:
- Evaluate severity in a systematic and consistent manner
- Coordinate care between local physicians and PH centers
- Treat contributing causes of PH aggressively
- Incorporate palliative care service in the management of PAH patients
- Participate in supervised exercise activity as part of the integrated care of their disease
- Maintain current immunization against influenza and pneumococcal pneumonia
- Avoid pregnancy. When pregnancy dose occur, we suggest care be provided at a pulmonary hypertension center
- Avoid exposure to high altitude. When exposure to high altitude or air travel occure, use supplemental oxygen as needed to maintain oxygen saturation >91%
- Avoid non-essential surgery. When surgery is necessary we suggest care at a pulmonary hypertension center

(Recommendation 1, 3, 6, 72-78; ungraded consensus-based)

↓

Suggest acute vasoreactivity testing at a center with experience
(Recommendation 7; ungraded consensus-based)

↓

Positive — **Treat with oral CCB**
(Recommendation 8; ungraded consensus-based)

Negative, RV failure or contraindication to CCB — **Should not be treated with oral CCB**
(Recommendation 9; ungraded consensus-based)

Figure 17.1 Treatment Algorithm for Pulmonary Arterial Hypertension (PAH) in Adults. *From Klinger JR, Elliott CC, Levine DJ, et al. Therapy for pulmonary arterial hypertension in adults. Update of the CHEST guideline and expert panel report. Chest. 2019;155(3):565–586.* Where multiple drug options are provided, there are no comparative effectiveness data to suggest greater benefit of one therapy over the other. *6MWD*, 6-min walk distance; *CCB*, Calcium channel blocker; *FC*, Functional class; *PAH*, Pulmonary arterial hypertension; *PH*, Pulmonary hypertension; *RV*, Right ventricular; *WHO*, World Health Organization. Refer to Reference 3 for recommendation numbers. * Combination therapy carries with it costs and potential for increased adverse effects and drug interactions. ** No data available for the oral/inhaled prostanoids use in whom parenteral prostanoids are indicated. *** Lung transplantation is outside the scope of this guideline and has not been evaluated by this panel.

Treatment-naïve PAH patients with WHO FC I → Continued monitoring for disease progression (Recommendation 4; ungraded consensus-based)

Treatment-naïve PAH patients with WHO FC II → Is the patient willing or able to tolerate combination therapy? *
- Yes → Combination therapy with **ambrisentan** and **tadalafil** (Recommendation 10; weak recommendation, moderate quality evidence)
- No → Monotherapy with either **bosentan, macitentan, ambrisentan, riociguat, sildenafil**, or **tadalafil** (See Box 1)

Treatment-naïve PAH patients with WHO FC III without evidence of rapid disease progression or poor prognosis → Is the patient willing and able to tolerate combination therapy?
- Yes → Combination therapy with **ambrisentan** and **tadalafil** (Recommendation 10; weak recommendation, moderate quality evidence)
- No → Monotherapy with either **bosentan, macitentan, ambrisentan, riociguat, sildenafil**, or **tadalafil** (See Box 2)

PAH patients with WHO FC III with evidence of rapid disease progression or poor prognosis → Is the patient willing and able to manage parenteral prostanoids?
- Yes → Continuous IV **epoprostenol**, IV **treprostinil**, or SC **treprostinil** (See Box 3)
- No → Consider addition of inhaled or oral prostanoid **

Determine when to start therapy

Figure 17.1 cont'd

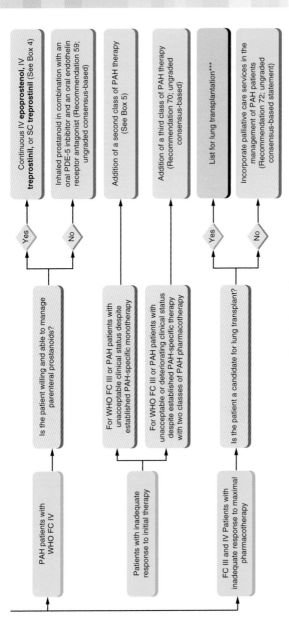

Figure 17.1 cont'd

Box 1: Treatment-naïve PAH patients with WHO FC II			
Drug	Outcome	Grade	Recommendation Number
Ambrisentan	Improve 6MWD	strong recommendation, low quality evidence	11
Bosentan	Delay time to clinical worsening	ungraded consensus-based statement	12–13
Macitentan	Delay time to clinical worsening	ungraded consensus-based statement	14
Sildenafil	Improve 6MWD	strong recommendation, low quality evidence	15
Tadalafil	Improve 6MWD	ungraded consensus-based statement	16
Riociguat	Improve 6MWD	ungraded consensus-based statement	17–20
	Improve WHO FC	ungraded consensus-based statement	
	Delay time to clinical worsening	ungraded consensus-based statement	
Parenteral or inhaled prostanoids should not be chosen as initial therapy or as second-line agent		ungraded consensus-based statement	21

Figure 17.1 cont'd

Box 2: Treatment-naïve PAH Patients with WHO FC III			
Drug	**Outcome**	**Grade**	**Recommendation Number**
Bosentan	Improve 6MWD	strong recommendation, moderate quality evidence	22
	Decrease hospitalizations related to PAH in the short-teram	weak recommendation, low quality evidence	23–24
Ambrisentan	Improve 6MWD	strong recommendation, low quality evidence	25
Macitentan	Improve WHO FC	ungraded consensus-based statement	26–27
	Delay time to clinical worsening	ungraded consensus-based statement	
Sildenafil	Improve 6MWD	Strong recommendation, low quality evidence	28–30
	Improve WHO FC	ungraded consensus-based statement	
Tadalafil	Improve 6MWD	ungraded consensus-based statement	31–34
	Improve WHO FC	ungraded consensus-based statement	
	Delay time to clinical worsening	ungraded consensus-based statement	
Riociguat	Improve 6MWD	ungraded consensus-based statement	35–38
	Improve WHO FC	ungraded consensus-based statement	
	Delay time to clinical worsening	ungraded consensus-based statement	

Figure 17.1 cont'd

Box 3: PAH patients with WHO FC III with evidence of rapid disease progression or prognosis			
Drug	**Outcome**	**Grade**	**Recommendation Number**
Continuous IV epoprostenol	Improve WHO FC	ungraded consensus-based statement	39–41
	Improve 6MWD	ungraded consensus-based statement	
Continuous IV treprostinil	Improve 6MWD	ungraded consensus-based statement	42
Continuous subcutaneous treprostinil	Improve 6MWD	ungraded consensus-based statement	43–44
For patients with continued progression of their disease, and/or markers of poor clinical prognosis despite treatment with one or two classes of oral agents, we advise consideration of the addition of a parenteral or inhaled prostanoid:			
IV epoprostenol	Improve WHO FC	ungraded consensus-based statement	45–47
	Improve 6MWD	ungraded consensus-based statement	
IV treprostinil	Improve 6MWD	ungraded consensus-based statement	48–49
In patients with PAH who remain symptomatic on stable and appropriate doses of an ERA or a PDE5 inhibitor, we suggest the addition of:			
Inhaled treprostinil	Improve 6MWD	weak recommendation low quality evidence	50
Inhaled iloprost	Improve WHO FC	ungraded consensus-based statement	51–52
	Delay time to clinical worsening	ungraded consensus-based statement	

Box 4: PAH patients with WHO FC IV			
Drug	**Outcome**	**Grade**	**Recommendation Number**
Continuous IV epoprostenol	Improve WHO FC	ungraded consensus-based statement	53–55
	Improve 6MWD	ungraded consensus-based statement	
Continuous IV treprostinil	Improve 6MWD	ungraded consensus-based statement	56
Continuous subcutaneous treprostinil	Improve 6MWD	ungraded consensus-based statement	57–58

Figure 17.1 cont'd

Box 5: Patients with inadequate response to initial therapy			
Drug	**Outcome**	**Grade**	**Recommendation Number**
In patients with PAH who remain symptomatic on stable doses of an ERA or a PDE5 inhibitor, we suggest the addition of:			
Inhaled iloprost	Improve 6MWD	ungraded consensus-based statement	61
Inhaled treprostinil	Improve 6MWD	strong recommendation, low quality evidence	62
In patients with PAH who remain symptomatic on stable doses of established IV epoprostenol, we suggest one of the following:			
Addition of sildenafil	Improve 6MWD	ungraded consensus-based statement	63
Up titration of epoprostenol	Improve 6MWD	ungraded consensus-based statement	
In patients with PAH who remain symptomatic on stable doses of bosentan ambrisentan or an inhaled prostanoid, we suggest the addition of			
Riociguat	Improve 6MWD	ungraded consensus-based statement	64–66
	Improve WHO FC	ungraded consensus-based statement	
	Delay time to clinical worsening	ungraded consensus-based statement	
In patients with PAH who remain symptomatic on stable doses of a PDE5 inhibitor or an inhaled prostanoid we suggest			
Macitentan	Improve 6MWD	ungraded consensus-based statement	67–69
	Improve WHO FC	ungraded consensus-based statement	
	Delay time to clinical worsening	ungraded consensus-based statement	
For stable or symptomatic PAH patients on background therapy with ambrisentan			
Addition of tadalafil	Improve 6MWD	ungraded consensus-based statement	71

Figure 17.1 cont'd

- Avoid in RV dysfunction, depressed cardiac output, or WHO Functional Class IV symptoms.

Targeted Therapies

Agents Targeting the Prostacyclin Pathway (Table 17.3)

- Mechanism of action (MOA): Prostacyclin produced in vascular endothelium causes potent vasodilation

Table 17.3 Agents Targeting the Prostacyclin Pathway

DRUG	EPOPROSTENOL IV FLOLAN	VELETRI	TREPROSTINIL IV OR SUBQ REMODULIN	TREPROSTINIL ORAL ORENITRAM	TREPROSTINIL INHALED TYVASO	ILOPROST INHALED VENTAVIS	SELEXIPAG ORAL UPTRAVI
Mechanism	Synthetic prostacyclin		Prostacyclin analogs	Prostacyclin analogs	Prostacyclin analogs	Prostacyclin analogs	A selective nonprostanoid prostacyclin receptor agonist
WHO-FC	III–IV	III–IV	III–IV	II–III	III	III–IV	II–III
Initial dose	2–4 ng/kg/min Titrate as tolerated Use IBW		1.25 ng/kg/min Increase by 1.25 ng/kg/min q7d; after 28 days, increase by 2.5 ng/kg/min q7d as appropriate Use IBW	0.25 mg q12h or 0.125 mg q8h Increase by 0.125 mg BID q3–4d	18–54 mcg QID	2.5–5 mcg 6–9 times daily	200 mcg BID Increase as tolerated to max 1600 mcg BID
Dosing: hepatic impairment	N/A		Mild-moderate: initial 0.625 ng/kg/min Severe: caution; titrate slowly Preferred route: SubQ	Mild hepatic: initial 0.125 mg q12h Moderate-severe: avoid	N/A	Moderate-severe: consider increasing dosing interval to q3–4h	Moderate-severe: initial 200 mcg daily, increase as tolerated Severe: avoid

$t_{1/2}$	6 min	4 h	4 h	4 h	25 min	Selexipag: 0.8–2.5 h; Active metabolite: 6.2–13.5 h
Stability	Protect from light; 8 h at RT; 24 h with cold packs	48 h at RT; 24 h at RT	—	Protect from light; 7 days once pouch opened	N/A; —	N/A; —
Adverse effects	Flushing, headache, N/V/D, jaw pain, thrombocytopenia		Flushing, headache, N/V/D, jaw pain, abdominal discomfort		Cough, throat irritation, bronchospasm, hypotension	Flushing, N/V/D, headache, jaw pain, muscle aches
Cautions	Abrupt discontinuation can cause rebound pulmonary hypertension (Applies to Epoprostenol, Treprostinil, & Iloprost)					CI: concurrent use with strong CYP2C8 inhibitors (i.e., gemfibrozil)

BID, Twice daily; *CI*, Contraindication; *CYP*, Cytochrome P450; *IBW*: ideal body weight; *N/V/D*, Nausea, vomiting, diarrhea; *RT*, Room temp; *SubQ*, Subcutaneously; $t_{1/2}$ Elimination half-life; *Temp*: Temperature

Data from Klinger JR, Elliott CG, Levine DJ, et al. Therapy for pulmonary arterial hypertension in adults. Update of the CHEST guideline and expert panel report. *Chest*. 2019;155(3):565–586.

and inhibits smooth muscle cell growth and platelet aggregation. A relative deficiency in prostacyclin production may contribute to the pathogenesis of PAH, and drugs targeting the prostacyclin pathway are one of the pharmacotherapeutic options for PAH.

Endothelin (ET) Receptor Antagonists (Table 17.4)

- MOA: ET-1 is a potent vasoconstrictor and promotes smooth muscle cell proliferation, fibrosis, and inflammation.

Table 17.4 Endothelin Receptor Antagonists

DRUG	BOSENTAN (TRACLEER)	AMBRISENTAN (LETAIRIS)	MACITENTAN (OPSUMIT)
WHO-FC	II–IV	II–III	II–IV
Receptor affinity	ET_A and ET_B	ET_A	ET_A and ET_B
Dosing	125 mg PO BID	5–10 mg PO daily	10 mg PO daily
$t_{1/2}$	5 h	9 h	16 h
BBW	Hepatoxicity and fetal toxicity; medication available only via restricted program under REMS	Fetal toxicity; females can only receive medication via REMS program	
Adverse effects	Hepatotoxicity, peripheral edema, and anemia		
	Most hepatotoxicity	Most peripheral edema	Most anemia
Drug interactions	CYP3A4 and CYP2C9 inhibitors and inducers; avoid cyclosporine and glyburide	Cyclosporine (max ambrisentan dose 5 mg daily)	CYP2C19 and CYP3A4 inhibitors and inducers

BBW, Black box warning; *BID*, Twice daily; *CYP*, Cytochrome P450; ET_A: Endothelin receptor type A; ET_B, Endothelin receptor type B; *PO*, Orally; *REMS*, Risk evaluation and mitigation strategy; $t_{1/2}$: elimination half-life; *WHO-FC*: World Health Organization Functional Class
Data from Klinger JR, Elliott CG, Levine CJ, et al. Therapy for pulmonary arterial hypertension in adults. Update of the CHEST guideline and expert panel report. Chest. 2019;155(3):565–586.

Abnormally high concentration of ET-1 has been found in patients with PAH. ET-1 exerts its action through two receptor subtypes of ET: ET_A and ET_B. Stimulation of ET_A and ET_B on smooth muscle cells leads to vasoconstriction, while ET_B stimulation may promote vasodilation and bronchoconstriction. Drugs selectively blocking ET_A receptors or by dual blockage of ET_A and ET_B receptors represent another class of pharmacotherapeutic treatment for PAH.

Phosphodiesterase Type 5 (PDE-5) Inhibitors (Table 17.5)

- MOA: PDE-5 in pulmonary vascular smooth muscle degrades cyclic guanosine monophosphate (cGMP) responsible for pulmonary vasculature relaxation. PDE-5 inhibitors work by increasing cGMP resulting in vasodilation in the pulmonary bed.

Soluble Guanylate Cyclase (sGC) Stimulator (Table 17.6)

- MOA: sGC stimulators work by increasing the sensitivity of sGC to endogenous nitric oxide (NO) and pulmonary vasodilator and by directly stimulating the receptors to induce vasodilation similar to NO.

Table 17.5 Phosphodiesterase Type 5 Inhibitors

| DRUG | SILDENAFIL | | TADALAFIL | VARDENAFIL (NON-FDA APPROVED) | |
	REVATIO (PO)	REVATIO (IV)	ADCIRCA	LEVITRA	STAXYN
WHO-FC	II–IV		II–IV	II–IV	
Dosing	IV 2.5–10 mg TID PO 20 mg q8h		40 mg PO daily	5 mg PO BID	
$t_{1/2}$	4 h		35 h	6–7 h	
Adverse effects	Headache, flushing, epistaxis, dyspnea, hypotension, and visual disturbance				
Drug interactions	Contraindicated in patients receiving nitrates; caution with CYP3A4 inhibitors/inducers				
	Dose adjustments with protease inhibitors, strong CYP3A4 inhibitors and inducers, CYP2C9		Cautious usage and monitoring with ritonavir	Dose adjustments with alpha-blockers and CYP3A4 inhibitors	
	Contraindicated with nitrates (Applies to Sildenafil, Tadalafil, & Vardenafil)				
Clinical pearls	Renal adjustments		—	Not yet indicated for PAH	

BID, Twice daily; *CYP,* Cytochrome P; *FDA,* Food and Drug Administration; *IV,* Intravenously; *PAH,* Pulmonary arterial hypertension; *PO,* Orally; $t_{1/2}$, Elimination half-life; *TID,* Three times daily; *WHO-FC,* World Health Organization Functional Class

Data from Klinger JR, Elliott CG, Levine DJ, et al. Therapy for pulmonary arterial hypertension in adults. Update of the CHEST guideline and expert panel report. *Chest.* 2019;155(3):565–586.

Table 17.6 Soluble Guanylate Cyclase Stimulant

DRUG	RIOCIGUAT (ADEMPAS)
WHO-FC	II–IV
Dosing	0.5–1 mg q8h (increase 0. 5 mg q14d as tolerated to max 2.5 mg) Smokers may require higher dose 0.5 mg TID with CYP and P-gp/BCRP inhibitors (i.e., azoles, protease inhibitors)
t$_{1/2}$	12 h
BBW	Fetal toxicity; females can only receive medication via REMS program
Adverse effects	Headache, stomach upset, reflux, dizziness, hypotension, N/V/D, constipation, anemia
Contraindications	Pregnancy, concurrent use with nitrates/nitric oxide donors or phosphodiestserase inhibitors (avoid if within 24 h of sildenafil or 24 h before or within 48 h after tadalafil)

BBW, Black box warning; *BCRP*, Breast cancer resistance protein; *CYP*, Cytochrome P; *N/V/D*, Nausea, vomiting, diarrhea; *REMS*, Risk evaluation and mitigation strategy; *t$_{1/2}$*: Elimination half-life; *TID*, Three times daily; *WHO-FC*, World Health Organization Functional Class
Data from Klinger JR, Elliott CG, Levine DJ, et al. Therapy for pulmonary arterial hypertension in adults. Update of the CHEST guideline and expert panel report. *Chest.* 2019;155(3):565–586.

References

1. Simonneau G, Robbins IM, Beghetti M, et al. Updated clinical classification of pulmonary hypertension. *J Am Coll Cardiol.* 2009;54:S43–S54.
2. Rubin LJ, American College of Chest Physicians. Diagnosis and management of pulmonary arterial hypertension: ACCP evidence-based clinical practice guidelines. *Chest.* 2004;126(1 Suppl):7S–10S.
3. Klinger JR, Elliott CG, Levine DJ, et al. Therapy for pulmonary arterial hypertension in adults. Update of the CHEST Guideline and Expert Panel report. *Chest.* 2019;155(3):565–586.

Miscellaneous

18

Acute Alcohol and Drug Poisoning

This chapter will review the pharmacotherapy for management of acute alcohol and drug poisoning according to the current practice guidelines by The American Academy of Clinical Toxicology and other expert panel.

INTRODUCTION

The primary treatment strategy for acute poisoning should focus on stabilizing the patient, with an emphasis on airway, breathing, and circulation.

MANAGEMENT AFTER PATIENT STABILIZATION

Gastrointestinal (GI) Decontamination

- To prevent the absorption of an ingested toxin from the GI tract
- Methods, indications, and contraindications (Table 18.1)

Acute Drug Poisoning

- Toxic syndromes (toxidromes) and specific therapies (Table 18.2)

Stimulants and Street Drug Overdose

- Toxidromes and therapies (Table 18.3)

Table 18.1 Gastrointestinal Decontamination: Methods, Indications, and Contraindications

METHODS	INDICATIONS	CONTRAINDICATIONS	DOSING
Activated charcoal (preferred)	Use within 1 h of ingestion of drug poisoning	Decreased level of consciousness or inability to protect airway Increased risk of gastrointestinal bleeding or perforation Recent bowel surgery Ingestion of acids, alkali, alcohols, carbamates, cyanide, organic solvents, hydrocarbons, metals, and organophosphates	Oral/NG: Single dose: 25–100 g Multidose: 50 g ×1 then 25–50 g q4h
Gastric lavage	Reserve for extraordinary situations involving life-threatening overdoses	Unprotected airway Increased risk of and severity for aspiration Ingestion of strong acid or alkali Increased risk of gastrointestinal bleeding or perforation	Lavage via large-bore OG tube with 200–300 mL of warm saline or water; continue until fluid is free of pills or pill fragments

Cathartics	Not recommended Conflicting data on decreased transit time in the GI track of drugs that are sustained-release, enteric coated, or poorly absorbed by activated charcoal	Bowel obstruction or perforation Absent bowel sounds Recent bowel surgery Volume depletion Electrolyte disturbances Renal insufficiency for magnesium citrate Hypotension	Sorbitol 70% solution 1–2 mL/kg or Magnesium citrate 10% solution 240 mL
Whole bowel irrigation	Not recommended for routine use May consider in potentially life-threatening ingestion of drugs with long half-lives, sustained-release, enteric coated drugs, or drugs that are poorly absorbed by activated charcoal (e.g., lithium, iron) May be useful in persons who ingest large quantities of illicit drugs for the purpose of smuggling (body packers)	Unprotected airway Ileus Recent bowel surgery Bowel obstruction or perforation Intractable vomiting Hemodynamic instability	Polyethylene glycol electrolyte solution 500–2000 mL/h until rectal effluent is clear

GI, Gastrointestinal; *NG*, Nasogastric; *OG*, Orogastric
Adapted from Frithsen IL, Simpson WM. Recognition and management of acute medication poisoning. *Am Fam Phys.* 2010;81(3)316–323.

Table 18.2 Toxic Syndromes and Treatment of Acute Medication Poisoning

DRUG	TOXIC SYNDROMES	TREATMENT
Acetaminophen	Anorexia; elevated liver enzymes; jaundice; pallor; lethargy; liver failure; N/V	Treatment based on Rumack-Matthew nomogram (see Fig. 18.1) N-acetylcysteine dosage: Oral (72 h): 140 mg/kg (LD), then 70 mg/kg q4h × 17 doses (MD) IV (21 h): 150 mg/kg (max 15 g) in 200 mL D5W infused over 60 min (LD), then 50 mg/kg (max 5 g) in 500 mL D5W over 4 h then 100 mg/kg (max 10 g) in 1 L D5W over 16 h (MD); reduce volume if weight <40 kg Limitations to using the Rumack-Matthew nomogram: presentation >24 h postingestion, unclear history of ingestion, overdose with extended-release formulations, chronic or repeated overdoses, preexisting hepatic disease, chronic alcohol use, or concurrent medications metabolized by the CYP system
Anticholinergics (antihistamines, antipsychotics, tricyclic antidepressants, skeletal muscle relaxants)	Agitation, hallucinations, abnormal movements, tachycardia, mydriasis, dry membranes, flushed/dry skin, hyperthermia, urinary retention, decreased bowel sounds	Physostigmine IV: 0.5–2 mg over 2–4 min, may repeat q0.5–1h PRN Benzodiazepines for seizures and agitation: lorazepam 1–4 mg IV push Avoid phenothiazines (e.g., chlorpromazine) and butyrophenones (e.g., haloperidol)

Benzodiazepines	Anterograde amnesia; ataxia; coma; confusion; drowsiness; lethargy; sedation	Flumazenil: 0.5 mg IV push; repeat 0.5 mg q1min PRN If no response 5 min after a cumulative dose of 5 mg, consider other causes of sedation CI: history of seizures, chronic benzodiazepine use, co-ingestion that could induce seizures (e.g., tricyclic antidepressants, cocaine) Propylene glycol toxicity from lorazepam or diazepam: characterized by hyperosmolarity and anion gap metabolic acidosis. Dialysis may be required for severe cases
β-Blockers (BBs)	Acidosis, bradycardia, bronchospasm, coma, hyper/hypoglycemia, hyperkalemia, hypotension, respiratory depression, seizures, prolonged AV conduction	Same treatment for BB and CCB: Atropine 0.5 mg IV push Glucagon 5–10 mg IV push; continuous infusion if symptom response achieved with bolus Calcium chloride 1–2 g or calcium gluconate 3–6 g IVPB; continuous infusion 0.3–0.7 mEq/kg/h if symptoms persist
Calcium channel blockers (CCBs)	Non-dihydropyridine CCB: hypotension, prolonged AV conduction, bradycardia, lethargy, hyperglycemia, and depressed consciousness Dihydropyridine CCB: vasodilation, hypotension, and reflex tachycardia	Norepinephrine 2–5 mcg/min, titrated to response Dopamine 5–10 mcg/kg/min, titrated to response Phenylephrine 20–40 mcg/min, titrated to response Hyperinsulinemic euglycemic therapy: Regular insulin 1 unit/kg IVP bolus (with dextrose bolus of 1 g/kg), then 0.5 unit/kg/h (with dextrose 0.5 g/kg/h) titrated until hypotension resolved or a maximum of 10 units/kg/h reached (keep serum glucose level at 100–250 mg/dL) Replete potassium PRN Sodium bicarbonate for QRS widening, severe acidosis, or dysrhythmia: 1–2 mEq/kg bolus; continuous infusion if symptoms persist

Continued

Table 18.2 Toxic Syndromes and Treatment of Acute Medication Poisoning—cont'd

DRUG	TOXIC SYNDROMES	TREATMENT
Clonidine	Apnea; bradycardia; coma; hyper- or hypotension; hypothermia; mental status change; pinpoint pupils	Naloxone: IV bolus: 0.04 mg then increase q2–3min to 0.5 mg, 2 mg, 4 mg, 10 mg, then 15 mg IV infusion: two-thirds the effective bolus dose per hour (0.04–4 mg/h) for patients requiring subsequent naloxone doses to sustain effect IV preferred, but can be given via endotracheal, intramuscular, intranasal, inhalational, intraosseous, or intrapulmonary route Atropine: 0.5–1 mg IV push Dopamine: 5–20 mcg/kg/min
Cholinergics (organophosphates, nerve agent exposure, physostigmine)	Hypersalivation, lacrimation, urinary/fecal incontinence, GI cramping, emesis, bradycardia, miosis, diaphoresis, pulmonary edema, weakness, muscle fasciculations, paralysis, bronchoconstriction	Atropine: 1–2 mg IV push ×1 then doubled dose q3–5min PRN until pulmonary muscarinic signs and symptoms are alleviated Pralidoxime (in addition to atropine): IV bolus: 30 mg/kg (max 2000 mg) over 30 min, then IV infusion: 8–10 mg/kg/h (max 650 mg/h)

Digoxin

Heart block, tachyarrhythmias, bradyarrhythmias, N/V, lethargy, headaches, confusion, and visual disturbances

Correct electrolyte abnormalities: K, Mg, Ca

Treat symptomatic bradyarrhythmias: atropine 0.5 mg IV push

Digoxin immune antigen-binding fragments (Fab) for life-threatening arrhythmias; asystole, VF/VT, complete heart block, symptomatic bradycardia, end-organ damage, hyperkalemia

Dosing:

If amount of digoxin ingested is unknown: 10–20 vials for acute toxicity or 6 vials for chronic toxicity

If amount of digoxin ingested is known: dose (vials) = [serum digoxin conc (ng/mL) × weight (kg)] / 100

Monitoring: serum digoxin concentrations are not recommended after the administration of Fab as a rapid rise in serum concentrations expected from the Fab-digoxin complex

Iron

N/V/D, hypovolemia, metabolic acidosis, seizures, hepatic/kidney failure, and GI tract scarring/strictures

Deferoxamine IV infusion: 5 mg/kg/h, titrate to 15 mg/kg/h as tolerated, max dose 6 g/day

Continued

Table 18.2 Toxic Syndromes and Treatment of Acute Medication Poisoning—cont'd

DRUG	TOXIC SYNDROMES	TREATMENT
Opioids	CNS depression, including coma, lethargy, or stupor; constipation, N/V; flushing and pruritus; hypotension; meiosis; pulmonary edema; respiratory depression; seizures	Naloxone: a competitive antagonist at the opioid receptor IV onset: 2 min; IV duration: 30–120 min IV bolus: 0.04 mg then increase q2–3min to 0.5 mg, 2 mg, 4 mg, 10 mg, then 15 mg IV infusion: two-thirds the effective bolus dose per hour (0.04–4 mg/h) for patients requiring subsequent naloxone doses to sustain effect IV preferred, but can be give via endotracheal, intramuscular, intranasal, inhalational, intraosseous, or intrapulmonary route
Salicylates	If serum concentration: <30 mg/dL: asymptomatic 15–30 mg/dL: therapeutic 30–50 mg/dL: hyperventilation, N/V, tinnitus, dizziness 50–70 mg/dL: tachypnea, fever, sweating, listlessness, dehydration >70 mg/dL: coma, seizures, stupor, hallucinations, cerebral edema, oliguria, dysrhythmias, hypotension, renal failure	No antidote for salicylate poisoning Gastric decontamination with activated charcoal for acute ingestions if the patient is alert without vomiting IV crystalloids to maintain BP IV glucose for hypoglycemia or significant neurologic symptoms Urine alkalinization to enhance renal elimination: 250 mL of sodium bicarbonate 8.4% over 1 h then 50 mL boluses PRN to maintain urine pH 7.5–8.5 or 150 mL of sodium bicarbonate 8.4% in 1L D5W at 2–3 mL/kg/h to maintain urine output 1–2 mL/kg/h to maintain urine pH ≥7.4 Replete serum potassium as necessary Consider hemodialysis if acute renal insufficiency, end-organ damage, altered mental status, deterioration of clinical status, or severe acid-base abnormalities

| **Sulfonylureas** | Coma, decreased appetite, dizziness, hypoglycemia, lethargy, seizures, weakness | Conscious patients: 8 oz of oral carbohydrate (juice, non-diet sodas, or milk) or oral glucose tablet/gel PRN BG <60 mg/dL
Unconscious patients: IV dextrose 0.5–1 g/kg q15min PRN BG <60 mg/dL
Octreotide: 50 mcg subcutaneous or IV q6h ×4
Glucagon: 1 mg IM, IV, or SubQ q15min PRN |
| **Tricyclic antide-pressants** | Coma; confusion; delirium; dilated pupils; dry mouth; seizure; hypotension; tachycardia; urinary incontinence | Benzodiazepines for seizures (avoid barbiturates and phenytoin): lorazepam 2–4 mg IV push
Sodium bicarbonate 1 mEq/kg IV push q15min until ECG stabilized or arterial pH goal (7.45–7.55) achieved
Dopamine 5–10 mcg/kg/min, titrated to response
Norepinephrine 2–5 mcg/min, titrated to response |

AV, Atrioventricular; *BG*, Blood glucose; *BP*, Blood pressure; *CI*, Contraindications; *CNS*, Central nervous system; *CYP*, Cytochrome P450; *D5W*, 5% dextrose; *ECG*, Electrocardiogram; *GI*, Gastrointestinal; *IM*, Intramuscularly; *IV*, Intravenously; *LD*, Loading dose; *MD*, Maintenance dose; *N/V/D*, Nausea, vomiting, and diarrhea; *PRN*, As needed; *SubQ*, Subcutaneously; *VF/VT*, Ventricular fibrillation or tachycardia

Adapted from Frithsen IL, Simpson WM. Recognition and management of acute medication poisoning. *Am Fam Physician*. 2010;81(3)316–323, and from Rasimas JJ, Sinclair CM. Assessment and management of toxidromes in the critical care unit. *Crit Care Clin*. 2017;33:521–541.

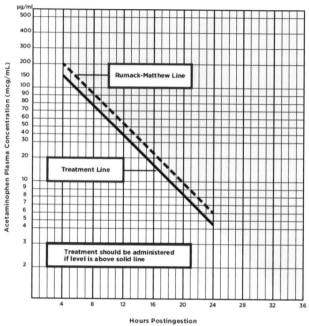

Figure 18.1 Rumack-Matthew Nomogram for Single Acute Acetaminophen Overdose. *Tylenol for Healthcare Professionals. Guidelines for the Management of Acetaminophen Overdose. McNeil Consumer Healthcare. www.tylenolprofessional.com/acetaminophen_overdose_treatment_info (1).pdf. Accessed July 30, 2019.*

Toxic Alcohol Poisoning: Methanol and Ethylene Glycol

- Toxidromes and therapies (Table 18.4)

Alcohol Withdrawal

- Clinical features (Table 18.5)
- Pharmacotherapy (Table 18.6)
- Monitoring (Table 18.7)

Table 18.3 Drugs of Abuse Poisoning: Toxic Syndromes and Treatment

DRUGS OF ABUSE	TOXIC SYNDROMES	TREATMENT
Amphetamines/ methamphetamines/ MDMA (ecstasy)	Confusion, tremor, anxiety, agitation, irritability, mydriasis, tachyarrhythmias, hepatocellular necrosis, acute hepatitis, myocardial ischemia, hypertension, cerebral hemorrhage, seizures, hyponatremia	Supportive care Gastric lavage or activated charcoal if within 1 h of ingestion Benzodiazepines for agitation Haloperidol or phenothiazines may be considered for patients with primary psychiatric disorders or dopamine-mediated movement disorders BP control with nitroglycerin, nitroprusside, or nicardipine. Avoid β-blockers because of unopposed α-receptor activity leading to an increase in BP
Synthetic cannabinoids: K2/spice	Euphoria or excited delirium, agitation, anxiety, hallucinations, paranoia, catatonia, cognitive impairment, ataxia, dizziness, headache, seizures, tachycardia, nausea; vomiting, palpitations, hypertension, acute kidney injury, rhabdomyolysis	Supportive care Benzodiazepines for agitation or seizures Haloperidol or phenothiazines may be considered for patients with primary psychiatric disorders or dopamine-mediated movement disorders

Continued

Table 18.3 Drugs of Abuse Poisoning: Toxic Syndromes and Treatment—cont'd

DRUGS OF ABUSE	TOXIC SYNDROMES	TREATMENT
Cocaine	Euphoria or excited delirium, agitation, anxiety, psychosis, delirium, stroke, subarachnoid or intracranial hemorrhage, seizures, tachycardia, palpitations, hypertension, arrhythmias, heart failure, aortic dissection, gastric ulcers, gastric perforation, bowel ischemia, status asthmaticus, pulmonary hypertension, pulmonary edema, alveolar hemorrhage, acute kidney injury, rhabdomyolysis	Supportive care Activated charcoal if within 1 h of oral ingestion Benzodiazepines for agitation or seizures; also effective for hypertension and tachycardia BP control with nitroglycerin, nitroprusside or nicardipine. Avoid β-blockers because of unopposed α-receptor activity leading to an increase in BP
Synthetic cathinones: bath salts	Euphoria, increased energy, and alertness, agitation, aggression, anxiety, paranoia, hallucinations, amnesia, confusion, insomnia, seizures, dizziness, headache, angina, hypertension, palpitations, tachycardia, abdominal pain, nausea, vomiting, anorexia, hepatic failure, AKI	Supportive care Benzodiazepines or antipsychotics for agitation or anxiety May consider propofol or dexmedetomidine for severe symptoms Antiemetics for severe nausea or vomiting

| **Piperazines** | Euphoria and increased energy, agitation, anxiety, hallucinations, psychosis, depressed mood, paranoia, confusion, insomnia, tremor, seizures, dizziness, headache, angina, hypertension, palpitations, tachycardia, QT prolongation, abdominal pain, nausea, vomiting, urinary retention | Supportive care
Benzodiazepines for agitation or seizures
Treat hypertension with IV antihypertensives or clonidine
Treat hyperthermia if temp >104°F (40°C) |
| **Ketamine** | Hallucinations and vivid dreams, impaired memory, cognitive dysfunction, severe agitation, hypertension, tachycardia, cardiac arrhythmias, laryngospasm, apnea, respiratory depression, anorexia, nausea, vomiting, cystitis, irritable bladder, urethritis | Supportive care
Activated charcoal if within 1 h of oral ingestion; may repeat q4h
Benzodiazepines for agitation or seizures; haloperidol if benzodiazepines ineffective |

AKI, Acute kidney injury; BP, Blood pressure; IV, Intravenously; MDMA, 3,4-methylenedioxy-methamphetamine; temp, Temperature
Data from Kersten BP, McLaughlin ME. Toxicology and management of novel psychoactive drugs. J Pharm Pract. 2015;28:50–65.

Table 18.4 Ethylene Glycol and Methanol Poisoning: Toxic Syndromes and Treatment

TOXIC ALCOHOLS	TOXIC SYNDROMES	TREATMENT
Ethylene glycol (main ingredient in many automotive antifreeze products)	Inebriation, altered mental status, nausea, vomiting, depressed consciousness, coma, generalized seizures, renal failure, pulmonary edema, and cardiovascular collapse	Fomepizole: preferred antidote MOA: competitive inhibition of alcohol dehydrogenase Dosing: 15 mg/kg IV bolus then 10 mg/kg q12h ×4; then 15 mg/kg q12h until methanol/ethylene glycol concentrations <20 mg/dL Hemodialysis increases the elimination of fomepizole; thus, change dose to 15 mg/kg IV q4h during hemodialysis Ethanol (if fomepizole unavailable) MOA: competitive inhibition of alcohol dehydrogenase IV must be compounded: dilute 95% alcohol Dosing: 10 mL/kg of a 10% solution, then 1.5 mL/kg/h until nontoxic. The goal is to maintain a serum ethanol concentration of 100 mg/dL (0.1%) until symptoms have diminished and methanol or ethylene glycol serum concentrations undetectable Hemodialysis: should be considered if clinical deterioration

| Methanol (common ingredient in shellac, varnish, windshield washer fluid, and solid cooking fuel) | Inebriation, visual disturbances, depressed consciousness, coma, and generalized seizures | Acidosis: Sodium bicarbonate 1–2 mEq/kg IV if pH <7.3
Seizures: benzodiazepines preferred
Adjunctive therapy:
Thiamine 100 mg IV daily
Pyridoxine 100 mg IV daily
Magnesium: 1–2 g IV ×1 if hypomagnesemia | Same treatment as ethylene glycol poisoning, except for the adjunctive therapy: folinic acid (Leucovorin) 50 mg IV q6h (if unavailable, use folic acid 50 mg IV q6h) |

IV, Intravenously; *IVPB,* ...; *MOA,* Mode of administration

Adapted from Rasimas JJ, Sinclair CM. Assessment and management of toxidromes in the critical care unit. *Crit Care Clin.* 2017;33:521–541 and from Miller H, Barceloux DG, Krenzelok EP, Olson K, Watson W. American Academy of Clinical Toxicology practice guidelines on the treatment of ethylene glycol poisoning. *Clin. Toxicol.* 1999;37(5):537–560.

Table 18.5 Clinical Presentation of Alcohol Withdrawal

FEATURES	ONSET AFTER LAST DRINK	DURATION
Early withdrawal (anxiety, agitation, tachypnea, tremulousness, tachycardia)	6–24 h	1–2 days
Seizures (generalized tonic-clonic)	6–48 h	2–3 days
Hallucinations (Visual, auditory, tactile)	12–48 h	1–2 days, up to 8 days
Delirium tremens (fever, tachycardia, hypertension, agitation, delirium)	48–96 h	1–8 days, up to 12 days

Adapted from Dixit D, Endicott J, Burry L, et al. Management of acute alcohol withdrawal syndrome in critically ill patients. *Pharmacotherapy.* 2016;36(7):797–822 and from Long D, Long B, Koyfman A. The emergency medicine management of severe alcohol withdrawal. *Am J Emerg Med.* 2017;35:1005–1011.

Table 18.6 Treatment of Alcohol Withdrawal

DRUG	DOSE	PK/PD	COMMENTS
Benzodiazepines: First Line			
MOA: bind directly to GABA_A receptor increasing the inhibitory effect of GABA on neuronal excitability			
Diazepam	5–10 mg PO/IV q6–8h PRN	Onset: 2–5 min (IV) Half-life: 43 ± 13 h Metabolism: hepatic (active)	Symptom-triggered dosing compared with fixed-schedule dosing shown to decrease total dosage and duration of treatment
Lorazepam	2–4 mg PO/IV q4–6h PRN	Onset: 15–20 min (IV) Half-life: 14 ± 5 h Metabolism: hepatic (inactive)	IM not recommended due to variable drug absorption
Chlordiazepoxide	50–100 mg PO/IV PRN, max 300 mg/day	Onset: 30–120 min (IV) Half-life: 10 ± 3.4 h Metabolism: hepatic (active)	
Oxazepam	15–30 mg PO q6–8h PRN	Onset: 120–180 min Half-life: 8 ± 2.4 h Metabolism: hepatic (inactive)	

Continued

Table 18.6 Treatment of Alcohol Withdrawal—cont'd

DRUG	DOSE	PK/PD	COMMENTS
Barbiturate: Second-Line if Benzodiazepines Inadequate			
MOA: potentiates synaptic inhibition by the GABA$_A$ receptor			
Phenobarbital	65–130 mg IV q15–20 min until symptoms controlled	Onset: 5min Half-life: 53–140 h Metabolism: hepatic	Off-label use; limited data Reserve for patients refractory to diazepam >150 mg or lorazepam >30 mg
α_2-Receptor Agonists: Off-Label Use			
MOA: activate an inhibitory neuron, leading to reduction in sympathetic outflow from the CNS			
Clonidine	0.1–0.3 mg PO q8–12h	Onset: N/A Half-life: 12–16 h (41 h in renal impairment) Metabolism: hepatic (inactive)	Helpful if catecholamine surge with elevated BP and HR Limited data
Dexmedetomidine	0.1–0.3 mcg/kg/h, up to 1 mcg/kg/h IV	Onset: 5–10 min Half-life: 6 min (terminal: up to 3 h) Metabolism: hepatic	Not recommended as mono-therapy; lack of GABA activity Helpful if elevated BP and HR

Selective GABA$_B$ Receptor Agonist: Off-Label Use		
Baclofen	10 mg PO q8–12h	Onset: N/A Half-life: 3.75 ± 0.96 h Metabolism: hepatic	Reduces signs and symptoms of alcohol withdrawal

GABA$_A$ Agonist and NMDA Antagonist: Off-Label Use		
Propofol	10–20 mcg/kg/min, up to 70 mcg/kg/min	Onset: N/A Half-life: 40 min (initial); 4–7 h (terminal) Metabolism: hepatic	Useful for mechanically ventilated patients refractory to benzodiazepines

Vitamins and Electrolytes		
Multivitamin	10 mL IV or one tablet daily ×3 days	N/A	Supportive care
Thiamine	100–500 mg daily ×3 days	N/A	Supportive care
Folic acid	1–5 mg daily ×3 days	N/A	Supportive care
Magnesium	1–4 g IV if hypomagnesemia	N/A	Supportive care
Potassium	10–40 mEq IV if hypokalemia	N/A	Supportive care

BP, Blood pressure; *CNS,* Central nervous system; *GABA,* γ-aminobutyric acid; *HR,* Heart rate; *IM,* Intramuscularly; *IV,* Intravenously; *MOA,* Mode of administration; *N/A,* Not applicable; *NMDA,* N-methyl-d-aspartate; *PD/PK,* Pharmacodynamics/pharmacokinetics; *PO,* Orally; *PRN,* As needed

Data from Dixit D, Endicott J, Burry L, et al. Management of acute alcohol withdrawal syndrome in critically ill patients. *Pharmacotherapy.* 2016;36(7):797–822 and from Schmidt KJ, Doshi MR, Holzhausen JM, Natavio A, Cadiz M, Winegardner JE. Treatment of severe alcohol withdrawal. *Ann Pharmacother.* 2016;50(5):389–401.

Table 18.7 Clinical Institute Withdrawal Assessment Scale for Alcohol, Revised (CIWA-Ar)

Nausea and Vomiting	Tactile Disturbances
0 No nausea or vomiting	0 None
1 Mild nausea without vomiting	1 Very mild paresthesias
2	2 Mild paresthesias
3	3 Moderate paresthesias
4 Intermittent nausea with dry heaves	4 Moderately severe hallucinations
5	5 Severe hallucinations
6	6 Extremely severe hallucinations
7 Constant nausea, frequent dry heaves and vomiting	7 Continuous hallucinations

Tremor	Auditory Disturbances
0 None	0 None
1 Not visible, but can be felt at fingertips	1 Very mild harshness or ability to frighten
2	2 Mild harshness or ability to frighten
3	3 Moderate harshness or ability to frighten
4 Moderate, with patient's arms extended	4 Moderately severe hallucinations
5	5 Severe hallucinations
6	6 Extremely severe hallucinations
7 Severe, even with arms not extended	7 Continuous hallucinations

Paroxysmal Sweats	Visual Disturbances
0 No sweat visible	0 None
1 Barely perceptible sweating, palms moist	1 Very mild photosensitivity
2	2 Mild photosensitivity
3	3 Moderate photosensitivity
4 Beads of sweat obvious on forehead	4 Moderately severe hallucinations
5	5 Severe hallucinations
6	6 Extremely severe hallucinations
7 Drenching sweats	7 Continuous hallucinations

Table 18.7 Clinical Institute Withdrawal Assessment Scale for Alcohol, Revised (CIWA-Ar)—cont'd

Anxiety	Headache, Fullness In Head
0 No anxiety, at ease	0 None
1 Mildly anxious	1 Very mild
2	2 Mild
3	3 Moderate
4 Moderately anxious, or guarded	4 Moderately severe
5	5 Severe
6	6 Very severe
7 Acute panic states as seen in severe delirium or acute schizophrenia	7 Extremely severe

Agitations	Orientation and Clouding of Sensorium
0 Normal activity	0 Oriented and can do serial addition
1 Somewhat more than normal activity	1 Cannot do serial additions or is uncertain about date
2	2 Disoriented for date by no more than 2 calendar days
3	
4 Moderately fidgety and restless	3 Disoriented for date by more than 2 calendar days
5	
6	4 Disoriented for place and/or person
7 Paces back and forth during most of the interview, or constantly thrashes about	

Total Score Is the Sum of Each Item Score (Maximum Possible Score 67)

Score interpretation:
<10: Very mild withdrawal
10–15: Mild withdrawal
16–20: Modest withdrawal
>20: Severe withdrawal

Adapted from Sullivan JT, Sykora K, Schneiderman J, Naranjo CA, Sellers EM. Assessment of alcohol withdrawal: the revised clinical institute withdrawal assessment for alcohol scale (CIWA-Ar). *Br J Addict.* 1989;84(11):1353–1357.

References

1. Frithsen IL, Simpson WM. Recognition and management of acute medication poisoning. *Am Fam Phys.* 2010;81(3):316–323.
2. Rasimas JJ, Sinclair CM. Assessment and management of toxidromes in the critical care unit. *Crit Care Clin.* 2017;33:521–541.
3. Kersten BP, McLaughlin ME. Toxicology and management of novel psychoactive drugs. *J Pharm Pract.* 2015;28:50–65.
4. Miller H, Barceloux DG, Krenzelok EP, Olson K, Watson W. American Academy of Clinical Toxicology practice guidelines on the treatment of ethylene glycol poisoning. *Clin Toxicol.* 1999;37(5):537–560.
5. Dixit D, Endicott J, Burry L, et al. Management of acute alcohol withdrawal syndrome in critically ill patients. *Pharmacotherapy.* 2016;36(7):797–822.
6. Long D, Long B, Koyfman A. The emergency medicine management of severe alcohol withdrawal. *Am J Emerg Med.* 2017;35:1005–1011.
7. Schmidt KJ, Doshi MR, Holzhausen JM, Natavio A, Cadiz M, Winegardner JE. Treatment of severe alcohol withdrawal. *Ann Pharmacother.* 2016;50(5):389–401.
8. Sullivan JT, Sykora K, Schneiderman J, Naranjo CA, Sellers EM. Assessment of alcohol withdrawal: the revised clinical institute withdrawal assessment for alcohol scale (CIWA-Ar). *Br J Addict.* 1989;84(11):1353–1357.

19

Anaphylaxis

This chapter will review the practice guideline on anaphylaxis by the American Academy of Allergy, Asthma, and Immunology and the American College of Allergy, Asthma, and Immunology.

INTRODUCTION

Anaphylaxis is an acute multiorgan dysfunction syndrome that may be potentially fatal if not treated promptly.

SIGNS AND SYMPTOMS (TABLE 19.1)

Table 19.1 Signs and Symptoms of Anaphylaxis[a]

Skin and mucosal tissue (most frequent)
- Hives, pruritis, flushing
- Angioedema

Respiratory
- Nasal discharge or congestion
- Upper airway angioedema
- Strider, shortness of breath, wheeze, cough, or bronchospasm

Cardiovascular
- Tachycardia
- Hypotension
- Dizziness
- Syncope

Continued

Table 19.1 Signs and Symptoms of Anaphylaxis[a]—cont'd

Gastrointestinal
- Nausea, vomiting, and/or diarrhea
- Abdominal cramps

Central nervous system (least frequent)
- Headache
- Seizure
- Feeling of impending doom

[a]Signs and symptoms listed in order of frequency

Adapted from Lieberman P, Nicklas RA, Randolph C, et al. Anaphylaxis—a practice parameter update 2015. *Ann Allergy Asthma Immunol.* 2015;115:341–384 and Simons FER. Anaphylaxis. *J Allergy Clin Immunol.* 2010;125:S161–S181.

TRIGGERS (TABLE 19.2)

Table 19.2 Triggers of Anaphylaxis

Immunologic mechanisms (IgE dependent)
- Foods such as peanut, tree nut, shellfish, fish, milk, egg, sesame, and food additives
- Medications such as β-lactam antibiotics, NSAIDs, and biological agents (monoclonal antibodies, allergens, vaccines, and hormones)
- Venoms such as stinging insects
- Natural rubber latex
- Occupational allergens
- Seminal fluid
- Inhalants such as horse, hamster, and other animal danders and grass pollen
- Radiocontrast media

Immunologic mechanisms (IgE independent; anaphylactoid reactions)
- Iron dextran
- Infliximab
- Radiocontrast media

Nonimmunologic mechanisms
- Physical factors such as exercise, cold, heat, and sunlight/UV radiation
- Ethanol
- Medications such as opioids
- Idiopathic anaphylaxis

Idiopathic anaphylaxis

IgE, Immunoglobulin E; *NSAIDs,* Nonsteroidal anti-inflammatory drugs; *UV,* Ultraviolet
Adapted from Simons FER. Anaphylaxis. *J Allergy Clin Immunol.* 2010;125:S161–S181.

ACUTE MANAGEMENT (TABLE 19.3)

Table 19.3 Acute Management of Anaphylaxis

I. Removal of offending allergen

II. Immediate treatment:
   a. IM epinephrine 0.3–0.5 mg, preferably in the mid-outer thigh. Repeat q5–15min PRN
   b. Place patient in recumbent position with lower extremities elevated unless contraindicated
   c. Protect airway
   d. Oxygen 8–10 L/min via facemask or up to 100% oxygen as needed
   e. 0.9% NaCl 1–2 L IV bolus. Repeat as needed
   f. Albuterol: For bronchospasm despite IM epinephrine, give 2.5–5 mg in 3 mL saline via nebulizer. Repeat as needed

III. Adjunctive therapies:
   a. H1 antihistamine: diphenhydramine 25–50 mg IV if urticaria/itching
   b. H2 antihistamine: Famotidine 20 mg IV (give with H1 antihistamine for additional relief of hives)
   c. Glucocorticoid (delayed onset of several hours): methylprednisolone 125 mg IV

IV. Treatment of refractory symptoms:
   a. Epinephrine infusion 0.1 mcg/kg/min, titrate q2–3min by 0.05 mcg/kg/min to blood pressure, heart rate, and oxygenation
   b. Vasopressors: in addition to epinephrine infusion as needed for blood pressure, heart rate, and oxygenation (see Chapter 12, Table 12.2)
   c. Glucagon: 1–5 mg IV over 5 min then 5–15 mcg/min for patients on β-blockers who do not respond to epinephrine

Note on epinephrine:
IM route into vastus lateralis is preferred due to:
• Rapid absorption reaching central circulation quickly
• Skeletal muscle well vascularized
• High risk of adverse effects by the IV route

IM, intramuscular; *IV*, Intravenous; *PRN*, As needed
Adapted from Lieberman P, Nicklas RA, Randolph C, et al. Anaphylaxis—a practice parameter update 2015. *Ann Allergy Asthma Immunol.* 2015;115:341–384 and from Simons FER. Anaphylaxis. *J Allergy Clin Immunol.* 2010;125:S161–S181.

PREVENTION[1,2]

- Avoid allergen or trigger
- Immunotherapy
- Desensitization
- Premedication

References

1. Lieberman P, Nicklas RA, Randolph C, et al. Anaphylaxis-a practice parameter update 2015. *Ann Allergy Asthma Immunol.* 2015;115:341–384.
2. Simons FER. Anaphylaxis. *J Allergy Clin Immunol.* 2010;125:S161–S181.

20

Drug-Induced Hyperthermia

This chapter will review the pharmacotherapy for management of drug-induced hyperthermia according to the expert opinion.

MALIGNANT HYPERTHERMIA (MH)[1,2,5]

Definition

A genetic disorder characterized by excessive release of calcium from the skeletal muscle resulting in muscle rigidity, hyperthermia, hypercarbia, and metabolic acidosis.

Triggering Agents

- Halogenated inhalational anesthetic (e.g., halothane, isoflurane, enflurane, sevoflurane, desflurane)
- Depolarizing neuromuscular blocker (e.g., succinylcholine)

Pharmacologic Management

- Initiate MH protocol and call MH hotline: 1-800-644-9737
- Discontinue Offending Agent(s)
- Dantrolene
  - Relaxes muscles by decreasing the release of calcium from the sarcoplasmic reticulum
  - 2.5 mg/kg intravenous (IV) push then 1 mg/kg until symptoms abate or a cumulative dose or 10 mg/kg reached

- To prevent recurrence: 1 mg/kg q4–6h ×24 h then 4–8 mg/kg/day divided into four doses ×1–3 days
- Avoid in advanced liver disease
- Treat Acidosis
  - Sodium bicarbonate 1–2 mEq/kg IV push over 5–10 min
- Treat Hyperkalemia
  - Calcium chloride 0.5–1 g IV or calcium gluconate 1–2 g IV over 5–10 min
  - Sodium bicarbonate 1–2 mEq IV push over 5–10 min (max 50 mEq per dose); do not give sodium bicarbonate in the same IV line as calcium
  - Insulin regular 10 units IV push with dextrose 50% 50 mL
- Treat dysrhythmias according to advanced Cardiovascular Life Support protocols
  - Procainamide has similar action to dantrolene and is thus drug of choice for MH-associated dysrhythmias
  - See Chapter 3.
- Calcium channel blockers in an acute MH crisis is contraindicated due to risk of worse hyperkalemia and hypotension.

NEUROLEPTIC MALIGNANT SYNDROME (NMS)[3]
Definition
An idiosyncratic drug reaction characterized by muscle rigidity, altered mental status, hyperthermia, and autonomic instability.

Triggering Agents
- Antipsychotic agents: haloperidol, clozapine, olanzapine, risperidone, phenothiazines
- Antiemetic agents: metoclopramide, droperidol, prochlorperazine
- Central nervous system stimulants: amphetamines, cocaine
- Other: lithium, tricyclic antidepressants

Pharmacologic Management

- Discontinue offending agent(s)
- Supportive care
- Benzodiazepines for agitation
  - Lorazepam 1–2 mg intramuscular (IM)/IV q4–6h or
  - Diazepam 5–10 mg IV q8h
- Dantrolene
  - Drug of choice for NMS
  - See MH for dosing
- Bromocriptine
  - A dopamine agonist
  - 2.5–5 mg orally (PO)/via nasogastric tube (NG) three times daily ×10 days after NMS controlled then taper slowly
  - Preferred over dantrolene in advanced liver disease
  - Can worsen psychosis and hypotension
- Amantadine
  - Dopaminergic and anticholinergic effects
  - Alternative to bromocriptine
  - 100 mg PO/NG twice daily (BID) up to 200 mg BID

SEROTONIN SYNDROME[4]

Definition

Overstimulation of serotonin receptors in the central nervous system characterized by mental status changes, autonomic hyperactivity (hypertension or hypotension, tachycardia, hyperthermia), and neuromuscular abnormalities (hyperkinesis, hyperreflexia, and clonus).

Triggering Agents

See Table 20.1.

Pharmacologic Management

- Discontinue offending agent(s)
- Supportive care
- Benzodiazepines for agitation: see NMS

Table 20.1 Serotonin Syndrome Triggering Agents

MECHANISM OF ACTION	DRUGS
Increase serotonin synthesis	L-tryptophan
Decrease serotonin breakdown	Monoamine oxidase inhibitors (e.g., linezolid) Ritonavir
Increase serotonin release	Amphetamines Methylenedioxy-methamphetamine (ecstasy) Cocaine Fenfluramine
Decrease serotonin reuptake	Selective serotonin reuptake inhibitors Tricyclic antidepressants Dextromethorphan Meperidine Fentanyl Tramadol
Stimulate serotonin receptor	Lithium Sumatriptan Buspirone Lysergic acid diethylamide (LSD)

- Cyproheptadine: antidote of choice
  - A serotonin antagonist
  - Initial dose: 12 mg PO/NG ×1 then 2 mg q2h until symptoms abate
  - Maintenance dose: 8 mg PO/NG q6h
  - May cause excessive sedation
- Chlorpromazine
  - Alternative to cyproheptadine
  - 50–100 mg IM q6h as needed

References

1. Larach MG, Gronert GA, Allen GC, Brandom BW, Lehman EB. Clinical presentation, treatment, and complications of malignant hyperthermia in North America from 1987–2006. *Anesth Analg.* 2010;110(2):498–507.
2. Malignant Hypothermia Association of the United States. https://www.mhaus.org/healthcare-professionals/managing-a-crisis/
3. Pileggi DJ, Cook AM. Neuroleptic malignant syndrome: focus on treatment and rechallenge. *Ann Pharmacother.* 2016;50(11):973–981.
4. Musselman ME, Saely S. Diagnosis and treatment of drug-induced hyperthermia. *Am J Health Syst Pharm.* 2013;70:34–42.

21

Fluids and Electrolyte Disorders

This chapter will review the pharmacotherapy for management of fluid and electrolyte disorders according to The Society for Endocrinology Endocrine Emergency Guidance and other expert panel.

GENERAL OVERVIEW (TABLES 21.1, 21.2, and 21.3)

HYPERNATREMIA[4]

- Defined as a serum sodium level >145 mEq/L
- Clinical manifestations: lethargy, irritability, restlessness, muscle spasticity, hyperreflexia, seizures, coma, and death
- Gross estimation of free water deficit (Adrogue-Madias) = $0.6 \times$ wt (kg) $\times$ [serum sodium/140 − 1]; use $0.5 \times$ wt (kg) for women. The Adrogue-Madias equation often underestimates total body water deficit.
- Dehydration: free water boluses using 200–300 mL q4–6h via feeding or suction tube. If no enteral route, intravenously (IV) as below

Management of Acute Hypernatremia (Hypernatremia ≤48 h): Rare

- Goal: decrease serum Na by 1–2 mEq/L per hour with max 10 mEq/L per 24 h
- 5% dextrose (D5W) IV @3–6 mL/kg/h until serum Na 145 mEq/L; monitor serum Na q2–3h

Table 21.1 Electrolyte Concentrations in the Extracellular and Intracellular Fluids and Daily Requirements

ELECTROLYTE	NORMAL SERUM CONCENTRATION	EXTRACELLULAR FLUID (mEq/L)	INTRACELLULAR FLUID (mEq/L)	DAILY REQUIREMENTS (g/DAY)
Sodium	135–145 mEq/L	142	10	1.2–1.5
Potassium	3.5–5.2 mEq/L	4	140	2.3–3.4
Chloride	95–105 mEq/L	103	4	1.8–2.3
Bicarbonate	24–32 mEq/L	28	10	N/A
Calcium	8.5–10.5 mg/dL	2.4	—	1–1.3
Magnesium	1.8–2.4 mg/dL	1.2	58	0.2–0.4
Phosphate	2.5–4.5 mg/dL	4	75	0.7–1.3

N/A, Not applicable.
Data from Hall JE. Guyton and Hall Textbook of Medical Physiology. Philadelphia: Elsevier; 2016: 47-59 (Chapter 4) and from National Academies of Sciences, Engineering, and Medicine. *Dietary Reference Intakes for Sodium and Potassium.* Washington, DC: The National Academies Press; 2019. https://doi.org/10.17226/25353.

Table 21.2 Electrolyte Composition of Intravenous Solutions

SOLUTIONS	SODIUM (mEq/L)	POTASSIUM (mEq/L)	CHLORIDE (mEq/L)	BICARBONATE (mEq/L)	CALCIUM (mEq/L)	MAGNESIUM (mEq/L)	OSMOLALITY (mOsm/kg)
5% Dextrose	—	—	—	—	—	—	252
0.9% NaCl	154	—	154	—	—	—	308
0.45% NaCl	77	—	77	—	—	—	154
5% Dextrose-0.225% NaCl	34	—	34	—	—	—	320
3% NaCl	513	—	513	—	—	—	1026
Lactated ringer	130	4	109	28	2.7	—	274
Plasmalyte, normosol	140	5	98	27	—	3	294

5% Dextrose, 5% Dextrose in water; NaCl, Sodium chloride

Table 21.3 Drugs that can induce Syndrome of Inappropriate Antidiuretic Hormone (SIADH)

DRUG	MECHANISM
Tricyclic antidepressants (e.g., amitriptyline, imipramine)	Increased hypothalamic production of antidiuretic hormone (ADH)
Selective serotonin reuptake inhibitors (e.g., fluoxetine, sertraline, paroxetine)	
Monoamine oxidase inhibitors	"
Phenothiazines (e.g., thioridazine, trifluoperazine)	"
Butyrophenones (e.g., haloperidol)	"
Antiepileptics (e.g., carbamazepine, oxcarbazepine, valproic acid)	"
Antineoplastic agents (e.g., vincristine, vinblastine, cisplatin, carboplatin, cyclophosphamide, ifosfamide, methotrexate)	"
Opiates	"
Antiepileptics (e.g., carbamazepine, lamotrigine)	Potentiation of ADH
Antidiabetics (e.g., chlorpropamide, tolbutamide)	"
Antineoplastic (e.g., cyclophosphamide)	"
Nonsteroidal anti-inflammatory agents	"

Adapted from Liamis G, Milionis H, Elisaf M. A review of drug-induced hyponatremia. *Am J Kidney Dis.* 2008;52:144–153.

- Once serum Na 145 mEq/L, decrease D5W to 1 mL/kg/h until serum Na 140 mEq/L
- Central diabetes insipidus: add desmopressin
  - Initial therapy: 5 to 10 mcg of the nasal spray every night (qhs)
  - 0.1 or 0.2 mg tablet qhs (may result in inadequate response)
  - 1 mcg subcutaneous q12h (if intranasal or oral route not feasible)
  - 2 mcg IV q12h (if inadequate response to subcutaneous)

Management of Chronic Hypernatremia (Hypernatremia >48 h): Common

- D5W IV @1.35 mL/h × weight (kg) to lower serum Na by max 10 mEq/L per 24 h
- If concurrent hypovolemia: 0.225% NaCl @1.8 mL/kg/h
- If concurrent hypovolemia and hypokalemia: 0.225% NaCl with KCl 40 meq/L @2.7 mL/kg/h
- Monitor serum sodium concentration q4–6h until goal achieved then q12–24h
- If hypernatremia due to correction of severe hyperglycemia and hypovolemia (e.g., diabetic ketoacidosis, hyperosmolar hyperglycemic state): 0.45% NaCl 6–12 mL/kg/h to lower serum Na by max 10 mEq/L per 24 h

HYPONATREMIA[5]

- Defined as a serum sodium level <135 mEq/L
- Clinical manifestations: lethargy, disorientation, restlessness, muscle weakness, depressed reflexes, seizures, coma, and death

Treatment of Acute or Severe Hyponatremia (Table 21.4)

- Hypervolemic: fluid and sodium restriction, diuretics
- Hypovolemic and low urine sodium: administer 0.9% NaCl IV or NaCl tablets 1–2 g three times daily
- Euvolemic:
  - Consider syndrome of inappropriate antidiuresis, secondary adrenal insufficiency, severe hypothyroidism, or drug induced

Table 21.4 Treatment of Acute or Severe Hyponatremia

INDICATION	TREATMENT	MONITORING	COMMENTS
If Serum Sodium <130 mEq/L			
Acute or chronic symptomatic hyponatremia (seizures, mental status changes, etc.) or known intracranial pathology (TBI, recent intracranial surgery or hemorrhage, etc.)	3% NaCl 150 mL over 20 min up to total 300 mL	Serum sodium q1h until serum sodium increased by 5 mEq/L	Acute hyponatremia: hyponatremia that developed over <48 h
Acute asymptomatic hyponatremia without autocorrection	3% NaCl 50 mL over 5 min; may repeat as needed		Chronic hyponatremia: hyponatremia ≥48 h or unknown duration Titrate 3% NaCl to increase serum sodium 5 mEq/L per day (max 10 mEq/L increase per day)

Continued

Table 21.4 Treatment of Acute or Severe Hyponatremia—cont'd

INDICATION	TREATMENT	MONITORING	COMMENTS
If Serum Sodium <120 mEq/L			
Chronic hyponatremia due to heart failure or cirrhosis	3% NaCl 15–30 mL/h plus IV furosemide BID (≥40 mg)	Serum sodium q2–4h until serum sodium increased by 4–6 mEq/L	Discontinue treatment if serum sodium ≥125 mEq/L
Chronic hyponatremia due to hypovolemia, adrenal insufficiency, or transient SIADH	3% NaCl 15–30 mL/h plus desmopressin IV/SubQ 1–2 mcg q6–8h		Titrate 3% NaCl to increase serum sodium 4–6 mEq/L per day (max 10 mEq/L increase per day)
High risk for osmotic demyelination syndrome			
Chronic hyponatremia other than above	3% NaCl 15–30 mL/h		

Note: corrected serum Na = measured serum Na + [(BG−100)/100×2.4]

BG, Blood glucose; *BID,* Twice daily; *IV,* Intravenously; *SIADH,* Syndrome of inappropriate antidiuretic hormone; *SubQ,* Subcutaneously; *TBI,* Traumatic brain injury

Data from Ball S, Barth J, Levy Miles, The Society for Endocrinology Clinical Committee. Emergency management of severe symptomatic hyponatremia in adult patients. *Emergency Guidance.* 2016;5(5):G4–G6.

- Fluid restriction and 0.9% NaCl IV
- If above measures inadequate, consider vasopressin receptor antagonists (Table 21.5)

Table 21.5 Vasopressin Receptor Antagonists for Hypervolemic or Euvolemic Hyponatremia

DRUG	STANDARD DOSING	COMMENT
Conivaptan (Vaprisol)	20 mg IV over 30 min ×1 then 20 mg over 24 h for 2–4 days, max 40 mg over 24 h	Avoid using >4 days Avoid in anuria or CrCl <30 Moderate-severe hepatic impairment: use with caution 10 mg IV over 30 min ×1 then 10 mg over 24 h for 2–4 days, max 20 mg over 24 h
Tolvaptan (Samsca)	15 mg PO daily, titrate at 24-h interval to max 60 mg daily	Avoid in liver disease, anuria, or CrCl <10 Avoid using >30 days Only initiate/reinitiate in hospitalized patients with close monitoring of serum sodium

CrCl, Creatinine clearance; *IV,* Intravenously; *PO,* Orally
Data from Jovanovich AJ, Berl T. Where vaptans do and do not fit in the treatment of hyponatremia. *Kidney Int.* 2013;83:563–567.

OTHER ELECTROLYTE ABNORMALITIES AND MANAGEMENT (TABLE 21.6)

Table 21.6 Electrolyte Abnormalities and Management

ELECTROLYTE ABNORMALITY SIGNS/SYMPTOMS	EMPIRIC TREATMENT	COMMENTS
Potassium (K)		
Hypokalemia: weakness, cramps, cardiac arrhythmias, flaccid paralysis, ileus	Serum K (mEq/L): 3.5–3.9: KCl 40 mEq IV/NG ×1 3–3.4: KCl 40 mEq IV/NG ×2 2–2.9: KCl 40 mEq IV/NG ×3 Infusion via peripheral vein: 10 mEq in 100 mL/h Infusion via central vein with continuous EKG monitoring: 20 mEq/h in 50 mL/h	Magnesium is a cofactor for the Na-K-ATPase pump, thus need to treat hypomagnesemia Use K acetate if acidosis Drug-induced hypokalemia: diuretics, amphotericin B, mineralocorticoid excess, piperacillin, ticarcillin, cisplatin
Hyperkalemia: EKG changes, symptoms similar to hypokalemia (weakness, paralysis)	Symptomatic or K ≥6 mEq/L: IV Ca gluconate 1–2 g or CaCl 0.5–1 g over 5–10 min IV regular insulin 10 units + D50% 25 g (omit if hyperglycemia) IV sodium bicarbonate 50–100 mEq IV over 5 min (if acidosis) Albuterol 10–20 mg nebulized Furosemide 20–40 mg IV Hemodialysis	NOT for acute hyperkalemia given delayed onset: Patiromer 4.2–16.8 g BID Sodium zirconium cyclosilicate: 10 g TID up to 48 h then 5–15 g daily Sodium polystyrene 25–50 g Drug-induced hyperkalemia: potassium-sparing diuretics, ACEI, ARB, NSAID, heparin, trimethoprim, octreotide, succinylcholine

Magnesium (Mg)

Hypomagnesemia: muscle weakness, cramping, paresthesias, Chvostek and Trousseau signs, tetany, QT prolongation, hypokalemia, hypocalcemia

Serum Mg (mg/dL):
1.6–1.8: 0.05 g/kg IV
1–1.5: 0.1 g/kg IV
<1: 0.15 g/kg IV
Max 8 g per administration
Infusion via peripheral/central vein: 1 g in 50 mL/h
Elemental Mg:
Mg oxide 400 mg: 19.8 mEq
Mg gluconate 500 mg: 2.2 mEq
Mg chloride 520 mg: 2.6 mEq

Drug-induced hypomagnesemia: diuretics, amphotericin B, caspofungin, foscarnet, cyclosporin/tacrolimus, pentamidine, aminoglycosides, piperacillin/tazobactam, cisplatin/carboplatin/ifosfamide/cetuximab, lactulose/orlistat, and potentially long-term use of digoxin or PPI
Oral Mg: adverse GI effects (e.g., diarrhea) makes it difficult to replenish in critically ill

Hypermagnesemia: hypotension, decreased deep tendon reflexes, bradycardia, somnolence, muscle paralysis, and arrhythmias generally do not occur until serum Mg >4 mg/dL

Symptomatic hypermagnesemia:
IV calcium gluconate 2 g over 5–10 min, repeat qih PRN
0.9% NaCl + loop diuretic
Hemodialysis

Drug-induced hypermagnesemia: magnesium antacids, magnesium citrate

Continued

Table 21.6 Electrolyte Abnormalities and Management—cont'd

ELECTROLYTE ABNORMALITY SIGNS/SYMPTOMS	EMPIRIC TREATMENT	COMMENTS
Phosphorus (Phos)		
Hypophosphatemia: weakness, paresthesias, seizures, coma, congestive cardiomyopathy, respiratory arrest, rhabdomyolysis	Serum phosphorus (mg/dL): 2.3–3: 0.16 mmol/kg IV 1.6–2.2: 0.32 mmol/kg IV <1.6: 0.64 mmol/kg IV Infusion via peripheral/central vein: 7.5 mmol in 100 mL/h	IV formulation: Kphos: 3 mmol phos + 4.4 mEq K Naphos: 3 mmol phos + 4 mEq Na PO/NG formulation: Neutra-phos and Neutra-phos K: 8 mmol of phosphorus per tablet/packet Drug-induced hypophosphatemia: insulin, catecholamines, antacids, sucralfate, Ca
Hyperphosphatemia: hypocalcemia, tetany neuromuscular irritability, prolonged QT; usually does not occur until Ca-phos product ≥55 mg/dL	Phosphate binders: Ca carbonate: 1 g QID Ca acetate: 1334–2001 mg TID Sevelamer: 800–1600 mg TID Lanthanum: 500 mg TID	Drug-induced hyperphosphatemia: vitamin D toxicity, phosphate enemas, bisphosphonates

Calcium (Ca)

Hypocalcemia: tingling, tetany, paresthesias, hyperactive deep tendon reflexes, Chvostek and Trousseau signs, prolonged QT interval, arrhythmia	Ionized Ca (mmol/L): 1–1.12: 2 g Ca gluconate IV in 100 mL NS or D5W over 2 h ≤0.99: 4 g Ca gluconate IV in 100–250 mL NS or D5W over 4 h Repeat until asymptomatic Ca chloride 1 g = Ca gluconate 3 g	99% Ca is in bone Highly protein bound in plasma Hypomagnesemia may impair parathyroid hormone secretion and end-organ resistance to parathyroid hormone Serum Ca concentration inaccurate in critically ill patients; use ionized Ca concentration Drug-induced hypocalcemia: amphotericin B, cisplatin, cyclosporine, foscarnet, bisphosphonates, loop diuretics
Hypercalcemia: mental status changes, polyuria, shortened QT interval, prolonged PR/QRS, muscle weakness, pancreatitis, bradycardia, atrioventricular block, renal impairment, nephrolithiasis	Serum calcium >14 mg/dL: IV NS 200–300 mL/h ×48 h Consider furosemide 40–80 mg IV q12h plus Calcitonin 4 units/kg IM or SubQ q12h, up to 8 units/kg dose plus Zoledronic acid 4 mg IV over 15 min or pamidronate 60–90 mg over 2 h	Calcitonin dosage forms: 200 unit/mL injection 200 units/actuation nasal spray Drug-induced hypercalcemia: thiazide diuretics, vitamin D Hypercalcemia due to some lymphomas, sarcoid, or other granulomatous disease: prednisone 20–40 mg daily Zoledronic acid, pamidronate: caution in renal failure

Continued

Table 21.6 Electrolyte Abnormalities and Management—cont'd

ELECTROLYTE ABNORMALITY SIGNS/SYMPTOMS	EMPIRIC TREATMENT	COMMENTS

Notes:

- Intracellular ions: recommend waiting 1–2 h after completion of the IV infusion before repeating labs
- Kidney is primary route of elimination for K, Mg, & phos
- Caution: CKD, AKI, ESRD, DKA, ongoing diuresis or GI loss, patient on parenteral nutrition, therapeutic hypothermia/targeted temperature management
- Consider decreasing empiric dosing by 50% if renal insufficiency

ACEI, Angiotensin-converting enzyme inhibitor; AKI, Acute kidney injury; ARB, Angiotensin receptor blockers; BID, Twice daily; CKD, Chronic kidney disease; D5W, 5% Dextrose; DKA, Diabetic ketoacidosis; EKG, Electrocardiogram; ESRD, End-stage renal disease; GI, Gastrointestinal; IM, Intramuscularly; IV, Intravenously; NG, Nasogastric; NS, 0.9% NaCl; NSAID, Nonsteroidal anti-inflammatory drug; PPI, Proton pump inhibitors; QID, Four times daily; TID, Three times daily
Adapted from Medford-Davis L, Rafique Z. Derangements of potassium. Emerg Med Clin N Am. 2014;32:329–347; and from Chang WW, Radin B, McCurdy MT. Calcium, magnesium, and phosphate abnormalities in the emergency department. Emerg Med Clin N Am. 2014;32:349–366.

References

1. Hall JE. Guyton and Hall Textbook of Medical Physiology. Philadelphia: Elsevier; 2016: 47-59 (Chapter 4).
2. National Academies of Sciences, Engineering, and Medicine. *Dietary Reference Intakes for Sodium and Potassium.* Washington, DC: The National Academies Press; 2019. https://doi.org/10.17226/25353.
3. Liamis G, Milionis H, Elisaf M. A review of drug-induced hyponatremia. *Am J Kidney Dis.* 2008;52:144-153.
4. Muhsin SA, Mount DB. Diagnosis and treatment of hypernatremia. *Best Pract Res Clin Endocrinol Metab.* 2016;30:189–203.
5. Ball S, Barth J, Levy M, The Society for Endocrinology Clinical Committee. Emergency management of severe symptomatic hyponatremia in adult patients. *Emergency Guidance.* 2016;5(5):G4–G6.
6. Jovanovich AJ, Berl T. Where vaptans do and do not fit in the treatment of hyponatremia. *Kidney International.* 2013;83:563–567.
7. Medford-Davis L, Rafique Z. Derangements of potassium. *Emerg Med Clin N Am.* 2014;32:329–347.
8. Chang WW, Radin B, McCurdy MT. Calcium, magnesium, and phosphate abnormalities in the emergency department. *Emerg Med Clin N Am.* 2014;32:349–366.

22

Pain, Agitation, Delirium, and Neuromuscular Blockade in the Intensive Care Unit (ICU)

This chapter will review recommendations from the 2013 Society of Critical Care Medicine and recently published research[1] (Fig. 22.1).

PAIN

- Greater than 50% of intensive care unit (ICU) survivors report significant pain during their ICU stay
- Common causes of pain in the ICU: acute trauma, injury or burns, postoperative pain, cancer pain, invasive procedures, and routine nursing care such as endotracheal tube suctioning, wound care, and tube insertion
- Short-term consequences of unrelieved pain: catabolic hypermetabolism, increased circulating catecholamines, impaired tissue perfusion, and decreased immune function
- Long-term consequences of unrelieved pain: chronic pain, lower health-related quality of life, neuropathic pain, and posttraumatic stress disorder
- Analgosedation: analgesia-first or analgesia-based sedation (treat with an opioid before a sedative)
- Assessment: assess pain q4–6h using either the Behavioral Pain Scale or Critical-Care Pain Observation Tool (Tables 22.1 and 22.2)
- Pharmacologic management (Tables 22.3 and 22.4)

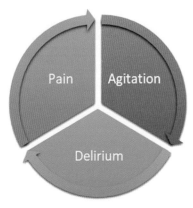

Figure 22.1 Pain, agitation, delirium.

Table 22.1 Behavioral Pain Scale (BPS)[a]

ITEM	DESCRIPTION	SCORE
Facial expression	Relaxed	1
	Party tightened (e.g., brow lowering)	2
	Fully tightened (e.g., eyelid closing)	3
	Grimacing	4
Upper limbs	No movement	1
	Partly bent	2
	Fully bent with finger flexion	3
	Permanently retracted	4
Compliance with ventilation	Tolerating movement	1
	Coughing but tolerating ventilation most of the time	2
	Fighting ventilator	3
	Unable to control ventilation	4

[a]A BPS score >5 indicates significant pain

Table 22.2 Critical-Care Pain Observation Tool (CPOT)[a]

INDICATOR	DESCRIPTION	SCORE
Facial expression	Relaxed	0
	Tense	1
	Grimacing	2
Body movements	Absence	0
	Protection	1
	Restlessness	2
Muscle tension	Relaxed	0
	Tense, rigid	1
	Very tense, rigid	2
Vent compliance	Tolerating	0
	Coughing	1
or	Fighting	2
vocalization	Talking normally	0
	Sighing, moaning	1
	Crying out, sobbing	2

[a]A CPOT score ≥3 indicates significant pain

AGITATION

- Identify and correct the etiology of the agitation
- Common causes of agitation in the ICU: pain, delirium, hypoxia, hypoglycemia, dehydration, and drug or alcohol withdrawal
- Light sedation, daily awakening trials, and minimal benzodiazepines recommended
- Assessment: assess level of sedation q2–4h using either the Richmond Agitation-Sedation Scale (RASS) or Riker Sedation-Agitation Scale (Riker SAS) (Tables 22.5 and 22.6)
- Pharmacologic management (Table 22.7)

Table 22.3 Opiates Commonly Used in the ICU

DRUG	USUAL DOSE	PD/PK (IV)	METABOLISM	COMMENTS
Fentanyl (Sublimaze)	Start at 0.5 mcg/kg/h Titrate by 0.25 mcg/kg/h q15min to CPOT <3 or BPS ≤5 Usual maximum: 5 mcg/kg/h	Onset: 1–2 min Duration: 0.5–1 h Half-life: 2–4 h	Hepatic CYP3A4 major substrate	Accumulates in hepatic failure Prolonged half-life with infusion duration Muscle rigidity <1%
Morphine	Start at 2 mg/h Titrate by 2 mg/h q15min to CPOT <3 or BPS ≤5 Usual maximum: 20 mg/h	Onset: 5–15 min Duration: 3–5 h Half-life: 3–4 h	Glucuronidation	Hypotension and bradycardia from histamine release Active metabolites, morphine-3-glucuronide (45–55%) and morphine-6 glucuronide (10–15%), accumulate in renal failure
Hydromorphone (Dilaudid)	Start at 0.25 mg/h Titrate by 0.25 mg/h q15min to CPOT <3 or BPS ≤5 Usual maximum: 2 mg/h	Onset: 5–15 min Duration: 3–4 h Half-life: 2–3 h	Glucuronidation	Accumulates in hepatic failure
Remifentanil (Ultiva)	LD 1.5 mcg/kg, followed by 0.5 mcg/kg/h Titrate by 0.5 mcg/kg/h q5min to CPOT <3 or BPS ≤5 Usual maximum: 15 mcg/kg/h	Onset: 1–3 min Duration: 3–10 min Half-life: 10–20 min	Blood and tissue esterases	Muscle rigidity >10% Rebound pain and withdrawal symptoms due to quick offset

BPS, Behavioral Pain Scale; CPOT, Critical-Care Pain Observation Tool; ICU, Intensive care unit; IV, Intravenously; LD, Loading dose; PD/PK, Pharmacodynamics/pharmacokinetics
Drugs without brand names are denoted by generic name only

Table 22.4 Non-Opioid Adjunctive Pain Medications

DRUG	USUAL DOSE	PD/PK	METABOLISM	COMMENTS
Acetaminophen (Ofirmev)	IV: 650 mg q4h–1 g q6h	Onset: 5–10 min Half-life: 10–20 min	Glucuronidation, sulfonation	CI in severe hepatic disease
Ketorolac (Toradol)	IM/IV: 30 mg then 15–30 mg q6h up to 5 days	Onset: 10 min Half-life: 2.4–8.6 h	Hydroxylation, conjugation/ renal excretion	Use with caution in renal/ hepatic dysfunction May increase risk of ARF, bleeding, or GI ADR
Gabapentin (Neurontin)	PO: 300–600 mg/ day÷2–3 doses	Onset: N/A Half-life: 5–7 h	Renal excretion	Renally adjust For neuropathic pain
Carbamazepine (Tegretol)	PO: 50–100 mg BID	Onset: 1–3 min Half-life: 25–65 h then 12–17 h	Oxidation	For neuropathic pain Caution in hepatic impairment Strong inducer of CYP enzymes, substrate of CYP3A4 ADR: SJS, TEN, pancytopenia, SIADH
Pregabalin	PO: 75–200 mg BID	Onset: days Half-life: 6 h	Urine (90% unchanged drug)	For neuropathic pain

| **Ketamine (Ketalar)** | IV: 0.5 mg/kg ×1 LD then 1–2 mcg/kg/min | Onset: 30 s Half-life: alpha: 10–15 min beta: 2.5 h | N-dealkylation, hydroxylation, conjugation | ADR >10%: confusion, irrational behavior, excitement, delirium, hallucinations For postsurgical patients to reduce opioid consumption |

Notes:
• Non-opioid adjunctive pain medications to be used in combination with opioids to reduce opioid use and optimize analgesia

ADR, Adverse drug reaction; *ARF*, Acute renal failure; *BID*, Twice daily; *CI*, Contraindication; *CYP*, cytochrome P450 enzymes; *GI*, Gastrointestinal; *IM*, Intramuscularly; *IV*, Intravenously; *LD*: Loading dose; *N/A*, Not applicable; *PD/PK*, Pharmacodynamics/pharmacokinetics; *PO*, Orally; *SIADH*, Syndrome of inappropriate antidiuretic hormone; *SJS*, Stevens-Johnson syndrome; *TEN*: toxic epidermal necrolysis

Table 22.5 Richmond Agitation-Sedation Scale (RASS)[a]

SCORE	TERM	DESCRIPTION
+4	Combative	Overly combative, violent; immediate danger to staff
+3	Very agitated	Pulls or removes tubes or catheters; aggressive
+2	Agitated	Frequently nonpurposeful movement, fights ventilator
+1	Restless	Anxious, but movements not aggressive or vigorous
0 (Goal)	Alert and calm	Alert and calm
−1	Drowsy	Not fully alert, but has sustained awakening to voice (>10 s)
−2	Light sedation	Briefly awakens with eye contact to voice (<10 s)
−3	Moderate sedation	Movement or eye opening to voice (but no eye contact)
−4	Deep sedation	No response to voice, but movement or eye opening to tactile stimulation
−5	Unarousable	No response to voice or tactile stimuli

[a]Sedation goal: RASS score of zero

DELIRIUM

- An acute and disturbed level of consciousness resulting in the inability to receive, process, store, and recall information
- May present as hyperactive (agitated and restless), hypoactive (flat affect, apathy, lethargy), or combination of both
- Associated with increased mortality, prolonged ICU and hospital length of stay, development of post-ICU cognitive impairment in adult ICU
- Assessment: assess delirium at least q8–12h using the Confusion Assessment Method of the ICU (CAM-ICU) or the Intensive Care Delirium Screening Checklist (ICDSC). Both CAM-ICU and ICDSC require a RASS (−3) or a Riker SAS (3) or more alert to be completed

Table 22.6 Riker Sedation-Agitation Scale (Riker SAS)[a]

SCORE	TERM	DESCRIPTION
7	Dangerous agitation	Pulling at ETT, trying to remove catheters, climbing over bed rail, striking at staff, thrashing side to side
6	Very agitated	Does not calm, despite frequent verbal reminding of limits; requires physical restraints, biting ETT
5	Agitated	Anxious or mildly agitated, attempting to sit up, calms down to verbal instructions
4 (Goal)	Calm and cooperative	Calm, awaken easily, follows commands
3	Sedated	Difficult to arouse; awakens to verbal stimuli or gentle shaking, but drifts off again; follows simple commands
2	Very sedated	Arouses to physical stimuli, but does not communicate or follow commands, may move spontaneously
1	Unarousable	Minimal or no response to noxious stimuli, does not communicate or follow commands

[a]Sedation goal: Riker SAS score of 4
ETT, Endotracheal tube

Table 22.7 Sedatives for Patients on Mechanical Ventilation in the ICU

DRUG	USUAL DOSE (IV)	PD/PK (IV)	METABOLISM	COMMENTS
Propofol (Diprivan)	Start at 5 mcg/kg/min Titrate by 5 mcg/kg/min q5min to RASS: −1 Max 50 mcg/kg/min	Onset: 1 min Duration: Short-term: 0.5–1 h Long-term: >7 days Half-life: Initial: 40 min Terminal: 4–7 h (after 10-day infusion, may be up to 1–3 days	Conjugation CYP2B6 substrate	Accumulation in severe hepatic impairment, cirrhosis, or with long-term infusion 10% lipid emulsion containing 1.1 kcal/mL; monitor TG Propofol-related infusion syndrome occurs at >50 mcg/kg/min for ≥48 h
Dexamedetomidine (Precedex)	Optional LD: 0.5–1 mcg/kg over 10 min Start at 0.2 mcg/kg/h Titrate by 0.2 mcg/kg/h q30min to RASS: −1 Max 1.5 mcg/kg/h	Onset: 5–10 min with LD 1–2 h without LD Duration: 1–2 h Half-life: 3 h	Glucuronidation and renal excretion CYP2A6 substrate	LD may initially cause severe tachycardia and hypertension, but can lead to bradycardia and hypotension A weak sedative with opiate sparing analgesic properties Sedative and analgesic properties, easily arousable, minimal respiratory depression

Lorazepam (Ativan)	1–4 mg q4–6h or 0.5 mg/h, titrate by 0.5 mg/h q30min to RASS: −1 Max 10 mg/h	Onset: 15–20 min Duration: 4–8 h, prolonged with continuous infusion Half-life: 8–15 h	Conjugation	Propylene glycol toxicity (HAGMA, nephrotoxicity) with lorazepam infusions for >48 h, at doses >6–8 mg/h
Midazolam (Versed)	1–4 mg q2–4h or 0.5 mg/h, titrate by 0.5 mg/h q30min to RASS: −1 Max 10 mg/h	Onset: 2–5 min Duration: 2–6 h, prolonged with continuous infusion Half-life: 3–11 h	CYP3A4 substrate Active metabolite	Lipid soluble Accumulates in hepatic/ renal dysfunction

Notes:
• Propofol or dexmedetomidine is recommended over benzodiazepines

CYP, Cytochrome P450 enzymes; *HAGMA*, High anion gap metabolic acidosis; *ICU*, Intensive care unit; *IV*, Intravenous; *LD*, Loading dose; *PD/PK*, Pharmacodynamics/pharmacokinetics; *RASS*, Richmond Agitation-Sedation Scale; *TG*, Triglycerides

- CAM-ICU
  - Diagnosis of delirium if 1 and 2 plus either 3 or 4
    1. Acute onset and fluctuating mental status
    2. Inattention
    3. Disorganized thinking
    4. Altered level of consciousness
- ICDSC
  - Eight components, each of which are allocated one point:
    - Level of consciousness
    - Inattention
    - Disorientation
    - Hallucinations-delusions-psychosis
    - Psychomotor agitation or retardation
    - Inappropriate speech or mood
    - Sleep-wake cycle disturbances
    - Symptom fluctuation
  - A score ≥4 indicates the presence of delirium
- Pharmacologic management (Table 22.8)

NEUROMUSCULAR BLOCKADE

- Assess the depth of neuromuscular blockade by peripheral nerve stimulators (e.g., Train-of-Four). Goals or paralysis can usually be reached with two or three of four twitches; zero of four twitches indicates complete neuromuscular blockade.
- Neuromuscular blocking agents (Table 22.9)

Table 22.8 Antipsychotics for Delirium

DRUG	USUAL INITIAL DOSE	PD/PK	METABOLISM	ADVERSE EFFECTS
Haloperidol (Haldol)	PO/NG/IM/IV: Elderly: 1–2 mg History of psychiatric disorders: 2–4 mg IV: non-FDA approved	Onset: IV, IM: 20 min PO: 2–6 h Half-life: 18 h	3A4, 2D6 substrates	Anticholinergic[a] Sedation[a] EPS[b] NMS[a]
Olanzapine (Zyprexa)	Start 5 mg PO/NG daily IM: resulted in unexplained deaths, may result in plasma concentrations 5× of oral administration	Onset: IM: 15–45 min PO: 6 h Half-life: 30 h	1A2 substrate Clearance increased by 40% in smokers and decreased by 30% in females	Anticholinergic[b] Sedation[b] EPS[a] NMS[a] Neuromuscular weakness
Quetiapine (Seroquel)	PO/NG: 50 mg 1–3 times daily Elderly: 12.5–25 mg	Onset: 1.5 h Half-life: 6 h	3A4 substrate	Anticholinergic[b] Sedation[b] NMS[a] Orthostatic hypotension[b]
Risperidone (Risperdal)	PO/NG: 0.25–0.5 once or twice daily	Onset: 1 h Half-life: 20 h	2D6 substrate	Anticholinergic[a] Sedation[a] EPS[b] NMS[a] Orthostatic hypotension[b] Cardiac conduction abnormalities

Continued

Table 22.8 Antipsychotics for Delirium—cont'd

DRUG	USUAL INITIAL DOSE	PD/PK	METABOLISM	ADVERSE EFFECTS
Ziprasidone (Geodon)	PO: 20 mg BID IM: 10 mg	Onset: IM: ≤60 min PO: 6–8 h Half-life: IM: 2–5 h PO: 7 h	1A2, 3A4 (minor) substrates	Anticholinergic[a] Sedation[a] EPS[a] NMS[a]

Notes:

- Incidence of QTc prolongation: IV haloperidol = ziprasidone > risperidone > olanzapine = quetiapine
- Antipsychotics
- Not recommended for prevention of delirium
- Reserve for significant distress and agitation harmful to patients themselves or others
- Recommend nonpharmacologic prevention of delirium such as sleep improvement and early mobilization

[a]Lower risk
[b]Medium-higher risk

BID, Twice daily; *EPS,* Extrapyramidal symptoms; *FDA,* Food and Drug Administration; *IM,* Intramuscular; *IV,* Intravenous; *NG,* Nasogastric; *NMS,* Neuroleptic malignant syndrome; *PD/PK,* Pharmacodynamics/pharmacokinetics; *PO,* Orally

Table 22.9 Neuromuscular Blocking Agents (NMBAs)

DRUG	USUAL DOSE	PD/PK	METABOLISM	COMMENTS
Depolarizing NMBA				
Succinyl-choline (Anectine)	IV, IM: 0.05–1.5 mg/kg	Onset: IV: 30–60 s IM: 2–3 min Duration: IV: 4–6 min IM: 10–30 min	Hydrolyzed by plasma pseudocholines-terase	Avoid in patients with a history of MH, stroke, hyperkalemia, paralysis, glaucoma, penetrating eye injuries, or spinal, crush, or burn injuries after 24 h
Nondepolarizing NMBA				
Pancuronium	IV: 0.06–0.1 mg/kg LD, followed by 0–2 mcg/kg/min	Onset: 3–5 min Duration: 60–120 min	Hepatic Active metabolite	Accumulation in hepatic/renal dysfunction ADR: vagolytic activity, sympathetic stimulation, bradycardia
Vecuronium (Norcuron)	IV: 0.08–0.1 mg/kg LD, followed by 0.8–1.7 mcg/kg/min	Onset: 3–5 min Duration: 30 min	Active metabolite	Vagolytic activity in higher doses
Rocuronium (Zemuron)	IV: 0.6–1 mg/kg LD, followed by 8–12 mcg/kg/min	Onset: 60–90 s Duration: 30–40 min	Minimally hepatic	Vagolytic activity in higher doses

Continued

Table 22.9 Neuromuscular Blocking Agents (NMBAs)—cont'd

DRUG	USUAL DOSE	PD/PK	METABOLISM	COMMENTS
Atracurium	IV: 0.4–0.5 mg/kg, followed by 4–20 mcg/kg/min	Onset: 2–3 min Duration: 20–40 min	Ester hydrolysis and Hofmann elimination	Histamine release
Cisatracurium (Nimbex)	IV: 0.15–0.2 mg/kg LD, followed by 3 mcg/kg/min Range: 0.5–10 mcg/kg/min	Onset: 2–3 min Duration: 30–60 min	Hofmann elimination	No histamine release

Notes:
- Reserve for patients with severe/refractory hypoxemia who fail conventional sedation and analgesia
- NMBAs must be combined with a sedative and an analgesic agent
- Consider using brain function monitoring such as Bispectral index (BIS)

Drugs without brand names are denoted by generic name only
ADR, Adverse drug reaction; *IM,* Intramuscularly; *IV,* Intravenously; *LD,* Loading dose; *MH,* Malignant hyperthermia; *NMBAs,* Neuromuscular blocking agents; *PK/PD,* Pharmacodynamics/pharmacokinetics

References

1. Devlin JW, Skrobik Y, Gelinas C, et al. Clinical practice guidelines for the prevention and management of pain, agitation/sedation, delirium, immobility, and sleep disruption in adult patients in the ICU. *Crit Care Med*. 2018;46(9):e825–e873.

23

Rapid Sequence Induction

This chapter will review the pharmacotherapy for management of rapid sequence induction outside the operating room according to expert opinion.

INTRODUCTION

Rapid sequence induction is the administration of an induction agent (anesthetic) and a neuromuscular blocking agent to rapidly produce unconsciousness and muscular paralysis to facilitate endotracheal intubation.

PHARMACOTHERAPY

See Table 23.1.

VASOPRESSORS FOR BLOOD PRESSURE SUPPORT

See Table 12.2.

Table 23.1 Pharmacotherapy for Rapid Sequence Induction (RSI)

DRUG	STANDARD DOSING (IV)	PHARMACOKINETICS	COMMENTS
Induction Agents			
Etomidate	0.3 mg/kg Shock: 0.15 mg/kg	Onset: 30–45 s Duration: 5–15 min	May suppress adrenal cortisol production; use cautiously in sepsis; consider hydrocortisone 100 mg IV ×1 Minimal hypotension; ideal for hemodynamic instability
Ketamine	1–2 mg/kg Shock: 1 mg/kg	Onset: 45–60 s Duration: 10–20 min	Beneficial in bronchospasm, septic shock, and hemodynamic compromise Minimal respiratory depression Causes catecholamine release, stimulant effects CI: elevated ICP or BP
Midazolam	0.1–0.3 mg/kg	Onset: 30–60 s Duration: 15–30 min	Amnesic properties Dose-related hypotension
Propofol	1.5–2.5 mg/kg	Onset: 15–45 s Duration: 5–10 min	Bronchodilation Respiratory depression, dose-related hypotension
Neuromuscular Blocking Agents			
Succinylcholine	1–1.5 mg/kg Use total BW	Onset: 30–60 s Duration: 5–10 min	Depolarizing NMBA Second dose can cause bradycardia (treat with atropine, see Table 3.1) NMBA of choice except for malignant hyperthermia, neuromuscular disease, muscular dystrophy, stroke or burn over 48 h old, rhabdomyolysis, significant hyperkalemia

Continued

Table 23.1 Pharmacotherapy for Rapid Sequence Induction (RSI)—cont'd

DRUG	STANDARD DOSING (IV)	PHARMACOKINETICS	COMMENTS
Rocuronium	1 mg/kg Use ideal BW	Onset: 45–60 s Duration: 30–45 min	Preferred nondepolarizing NMBAs due to shorter onset and duration compared to other agents in the same class
Vecuronium	0.1 mg/kg	Onset: 3–4 min Duration: 35–45 min	Alternative nondepolarizing NMBA to rocuronium

Notes:
- Pancuronium is not recommended due to tachycardia and histamine release and longer onset and duration compared to other NMBAs
- Sugammadex:
  - A reversal agent for rocuronium and vecuronium; a rescue agent if unable to intubate/ventilate
  - Routine reversal of rocuronium or vecuronium: 2–4 mg/kg
  - Immediate reversal of rocuronium: 16 mg/kg
  - Risk of bradycardia: monitor electrocardiogram
  - Risk of anaphylaxis: have resuscitation drugs readily available
  - Use not recommended in CrCl <30 and dialysis

- Neostimine
  - A reversal agent for nondepolarizing NMBAs
  - Only give when there is adequate recovery (train-of-four ≥10% of baseline)
  - Dose: 0.05–0.07 mg/kg IV ×1
  - Glycopyrrolate IV (0.2 mg for each 1 mg of neostigmine) should be given prior to or in conjunction with neostigmine

BP, Blood pressure; *BW*, Body weight; *CI*, Contraindication; *CrCl*, Creatinine clearance; *ICP*, Intracranial pressure; *IV*, Intravenous; *NMBA*, Neuromuscular blocking agent

Data from Mosier JM, Sakles JC, Stolz U, et al. Neuromuscular blockade improves first-attempt success for intubation in the intensive care unit: a propensity matched analysis. *Ann Am Thorac Soc.* 2015;12(5):734–741; and from Sakles JC, Douglas MJK, Hypes CD, et al. Management of patients with predicted difficult airways in an academic emergency department. *J Emergency Med.* 2017;53(2):163–171.

References

1. Mosier JM, Sakles JC, Stolz U, et al. Neuromuscular blockade improves first-attempt success for intubation in the intensive care unit: a propensity matched analysis. *Ann Am Thorac Soc.* 2015;12(5):734–741.
2. Sakles JC, Douglas MJK, Hypes CD, Patanwala AE, Mosier JM. Management of patients with predicted difficult airways in an academic emergency department. *J Emergency Med.* 2017;53(2):163–171.

24

Venous Thromboembolism (VTE)

This chapter will review the pharmacotherapy for prevention and treatment of venous thromboembolism according to the American College of Chest Physicians evidence-based clinical practice guidelines on antithrombotic therapy and prevention of thrombosis.

INTRODUCTION

The threat of pulmonary embolism (PE) is a daily concern for patients in the intensive care unit (ICU), who typically have one or more risk factors for venous thromboembolism (VTE), the precursor of pulmonary embolism.

RISK FACTORS FOR VTE

See Table 24.1.

PREVALENCE OF VTE

See Fig. 24.1.

THROMBOPROPHYLAXIS

- Thromboprophylaxis for specific conditions (Table 24.2)
- Pharmacotherapy according to specific conditions (Table 24.3)

Table 24.1 Risk Factors for VTE in Hospitalized Patients

Surgery	Major surgery, especially cancer-related surgery, hip and knee surgery
Trauma	Multisystem trauma, especially spinal cord injury and fractures of the spine
Malignancy	Any malignancy, active or occult chemotherapy and radiotherapy
Acute medical illness	Stroke, right-sided heart failure, sepsis, inflammatory bowel disease, nephrotic syndrome, myeloproliferative disorders
Drugs	Erythropoiesis-stimulating drugs, estrogen-containing compounds
Patient-specific factors	Prior thromboembolism, obesity, increasing age, pregnancy
ICU-related factors	Prolonged mechanical ventilation, neuromuscular paralysis, severe sepsis, vasopressors, platelet transfusions, immobility

ICU, Intensive care unit; *VTE,* Venous thromboembolism
Data from Goldhaber SZ. Risk factors for venous thromboembolism. *J Am Coll Cardiol.* 2010;56(1):1–7; and Lijfering WM, Rosendaal FR, Cannegieter SC. Risk factors for venous thrombosis—current understanding from an epidemiological point of view. *Br J Haematol.* 2010;149(6):824–833.

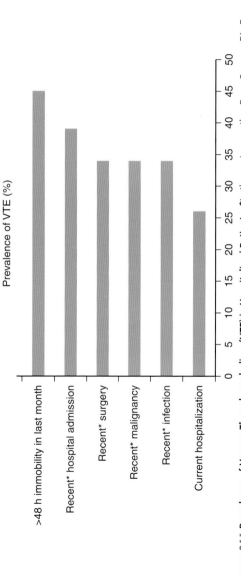

Figure 24.1 Prevalence of Venous Thromboembolism (VTE) in Hospitalized Patients. *In the past 3 months. From Spencer FA, Emery C, Lessard D, et al. The Worcester Venous Thromboembolism Study: a population-based study of the clinical epidemiology of venous thromboembolism. J Gen Intern Med. 2006;21:722–727.*

Table 24.2 Thromboprophylaxis for Specific Conditions

CONDITIONS	REGIMENS (ANY DRUG OR MECHANICAL DEVICE)								
	UFH	LMWH	FONDAPARINUX	ASA	APIXABAN	DABIGATRAN	RIVAROXABAN	WARFARIN	IPC
Acute medical illness	+	+	+						
General and abdominal-pelvic surgery									
Low risk	+	+							+
Moderate risk	+	+							+
High risk	+	+	+[a]	+[a]					+[b]
Abdominal-pelvic surgery for cancer	+	+							
Thoracic Surgery									
Moderate risk	+	+							+
High risk	+	+							+[b]
Cardiac surgery with complications	+	+							+[b]
Craniotomy	+	+							+
Spinal surgery	+	+							+
Hip or knee surgery	+[c]	+	+[c]	+[c]	+[c]	+[c]	+[c]	+[c]	+[c]

Major orthopedic surgery			+	+	+[d]	+[e]
Major trauma	+	+	+			+
Head or spinal cord injury	+	+			+[d]	+[b]
Any of the above + active bleeding or high risk of bleeding						+

[a]If contraindicated to *UFH* or *LMWH*
[b]Combined with *UFH* or *LMWH*
[c]Alternative (*LMWH*, Preferred)
[d]Second-line agent
[e]Combined with apixaban or dabigatran

ASA, Aspirin; IPC, Intermittent pneumatic compression; LMWH, Low-molecular-weight heparin; UFH, Unfractionated heparin
Data from Falck-Ytter Y, Francis CW, Johanson NA, et al. Prevention of VTE in orthopedic surgery patients. *Chest*. 2012;141(2 suppl):e278S–e325S; and Gould MK, Garcia DA, Wren SM, et al. Prevention of VTE in nonorthopedic surgical patients. *Chest*. 2012;141(2 suppl):e227S–e277S.

Table 24.3 Pharmacotherapy for Thromboprophylaxis According to Specific Conditions[a]

ANTICOAGULANT	USUAL DOSE	DOSE ADJUSTMENT	COMMENTS
Unfractionated Heparin			
UFH	5000 units SubQ q8–12h	BMI ≥50: 7000 units q8h	LWMH has a lower risk of HIT compared to UFH
Low-Molecular-Weight Heparins			
Enoxaparin	40 mg SubQ q24h or 30 mg SubQ q12h	BMI >40: 0.5 mg/kg q24h CrCl <30: 30 mg q24h	LMWH is equivalent to UFH for most conditions in ICU except for orthopedic procedures involving the hip and knee (LMWH is superior to UFH)
Dalteparin	2500–5000 units SubQ q24h	No adjustment	First dose of LMWH should not be given <12 h after surgery
Factor Xa Inhibitors			
Fondaparinux	2.5 mg SubQ q24h	CI: <50 kg or CrCl <30: avoid	Useful for patients with history of HIT
Betrixaban (Bevyxxa)	160 mg ×1 then 80 mg PO daily with food ×35–42 days	CrCl 15–29 or strong P-gp inhibitors (e.g., amiodarone, azithromycin, clarithromycin, ketoconazole, verapamil): 80 mg ×1 then 40 mg PO daily with food ×35–42 days CrCl <15 or dialysis: not studied	New prophylactic anticoagulant for acute medical illness

Antiplatelet			
Aspirin	160 mg PO daily	Caution in CrCl <10	N/A
Direct Oral Anticoagulants			
Apixaban	2.5 mg PO BID	CrCl <30: excluded from studies	Apixaban, dabigatran, and rivaroxaban can elevate the INR
Dabigatran	150 mg–220 mg PO daily	CrCl ≤30: excluded from studies	
Rivaroxaban	10 mg PO daily	CrCl <30: avoid	
Vitamin K Antagonist			
Warfarin	5–10 mg PO daily for 2 days, then titrate to INR 2–3	Monitor INR closely	Monitor INR closely

*Refer to specific conditions in Table 24.2

BID, Twice daily; *BMI*, Body mass index; *CI*, Contraindicated; *CrCl*, Creatinine clearance; *HIT*, Heparin-induced thrombocytopenia; *ICU*, Intensive care unit; *INR*, International normalized ratio; *LMWH*, Low-molecular-weight heparin; *P-gp*, P-glycoprotein; *PO*, Orally; *SubQ*, Subcutaneous; *UFH*, Unfractionated heparin

From Guyatt GH, Akl EA, Crowther M, et al. Executive summary antithrombotic therapy and prevention of thrombosis, 9th ed: American College of Chest Physicians evidence-based clinical practice guidelines. *Chest.* 2012;141(2 suppl):7S–47S.

Table 24.4 Sample of Weight-Based Heparin Dosing Regimen

1. Give initial bolus 80 units/kg then continuous infusion 18 units/kg/h
   Use adjusted body weight when patient is obese (≥20% above IBW)
   Adjusted weight (kg) = IBW + 0.4 × (actual weight − IBW)
   Men: IBW (kg) = 50 + 2.3 × (height >60 inches)
   Women: IBW (kg) = 45 + 2.3 × (height >60 inches)

2. Check aPTT 6 h after start of infusion and adjust heparin dose as below

aPTT (s) [a]	BOLUS DOSE	HOLD INFUSION	CONTINUOUS INFUSION
<35	80 units/kg	—	↑ by 4 units/kg/h
35–49	40 units/kg	—	↑ by 2 units/kg/h
50–84 (goal)	—	—	—
85–105	—	—	↓ by 2 units/kg/h
106–140	—	Hold for 1 h	↓ by 3 units/kg/h
>140	Hold and repeat aPTT q2h until aPTT <140		

3. Check aPTT 6 h after each dose adjustment. When aPTT at goal, monitor daily

[a] aPTT, based on control value 29 s, aPTT goal and titration variable depending institution
aPTT, Activated partial thromboplastin time; *IBW*, Ideal body weight; *s*, Seconds
From Holbrook A, Schulman s, Witt DM, et al. Evidence-based management of anticoagulant therapy: antithrombotic therapy and prevention of thrombosis, 9th ed: American College of Chest Physicians evidence-based clinical practice guidelines. *Chest.* 2012;141(2 suppl): e152S–e184S.

TREATMENT OF VTE WITH ANTICOAGULANTS

- Unfractionated heparin (UFH): preferred in the intensive care unit (ICU) because it is rapidly acting, can be reversed promptly with protamine, and does not require renal dosing (Table 24.4).
- Low-molecular-weight heparin (LMWH) (Table 24.5)
  - More appropriate for non-ICU patients and outpatients
  - Preferred long-term treatment for VTE and cancer
- New oral anticoagulants (Table 24.6)
  - Preferred over warfarin
- Warfarin (1, 2, 2.5, 3, 4, 5, 6, 7.5, 10 mg tablets)
  - Preferred over LMWH if VTE and *no* cancer

Table 24.5 Therapeutic LMWH

DRUG FORM	STANDARD DOSING (SubQ) USE ACTUAL WEIGHT	DOSE ADJUSTMENT
Dalteparin (Fragmin) 2500 units/0.2 mL, 5000 units/0.2 mL, 7500 units/0.3 mL, 10,000 units/mL, 12,500 units/0.5 mL, 15,000 units/0.6 mL, 18,000 units/0.72 mL	200 units/kg daily ×30 days then 150 units/kg daily ×2–6 months[a]; max 18,000 units/dose	Platelet 50,000–100,000: decrease dose by 2500 units if 46-82 kg and by 3000 units if ≥83 kg Platelet <50,000: discontinue
Enoxaparin (Lovenox) 30 mg/0.3 mL, 40 mg/0.4 mL, 60 mg/ 0.6 mL, 80 mg/0.8 mL, 100 mg/mL, 120 mg/0.8 mL, 150 mg/mL	1 mg/kg q12h (preferred) or 1.5 mg/kg q24h	CrCl <30: 1 mg/kg q24h Not FDA approved for use in dialysis
Tinzaparin (Innohep) 2500 units/0.25 mL, 3500 units/0.35 mL, 4500 units/0.45 mL, 8000 units/0.4 mL, 10,000 units/0.5 mL, 12,000 units/0.6 mL, 14,000 units/0.7 mL, 16,000 units/0.8 mL, 18,000 units/0.9 mL Not available in U.S.	175 anti-Xa units/kg q24h Max: 18,000 anti-Xa units/day	CrCl <30: use with caution Not dialyzable

Continued

Table 24.5 Therapeutic LMWH—cont'd

DRUG FORM	STANDARD DOSING (SubQ) USE ACTUAL WEIGHT	DOSE ADJUSTMENT
Nadroparin (Fraxiparine) 9500 units/mL (0.3 mL, 0.4 mL, 0.6 mL, 1 mL) (Fraxiparine Forte) 19,000 units/mL (0.6 mL, 0.8 mL, 1 mL) Not available in U.S.	No increased risk for bleeding: 171 units/kg once daily Increased risk for bleeding: 86 units/kg q12h Max: 17,100 units/day	CrCl 30–49: decrease dose by 25–33% CrCl <30: avoid use Not dialyzable

aDosing for venous thromboembolism treatment with active cancer

CrCl, Creatinine clearance; FDA, Food and Drug Administration; LMWH, Low-molecular-weight heparin; max, Maximum; SubQ, Subcutaneous

From Holbrook A, Schulman s, Witt DM, et al. Evidence-based management of anticoagulant therapy: antithrombotic therapy and prevention of thrombosis, 9th ed: American College of Chest Physicians evidence-based clinical practice guidelines. Chest. 2012;141(2 suppl):e152S–e184S.

Table 24.6 Direct Oral Anticoagulants (DOACs)

DRUG FORM	STANDARD DOSING	RENAL DOSING (USE ACTUAL WEIGHT FOR CrCl)	DRUG INTERACTION
Apixaban (Eliquis) 2.5 mg, 5 mg	10 mg BID ×7 days, then 5 mg BID After 6 months: 2.5 mg BID	Not dialyzable	Avoid use with combined CYP3A4 and P-gp inducers (e.g., rifampin, phenytoin, carbamazepine, St. John's wort) Combined strong CYP3A4 and P-gp inhibitors: reduce dose by 50%. If patient already on reduced dose, then avoid concurrent use
Dabigatran (Pradaxa) 75 mg, 110 mg, 150 mg	Following 5–10 days of parenteral anticoagulant, begin dabigatran 150 mg BID	CrCl <50 and concomitant P-gp inhibitors: avoid use Crcl <30: avoid use	Avoid use with P-gp inducers (e.g., rifampin)
Edoxaban (Savaysa) 15 mg, 30 mg, 60 mg	Following 5–10 days of parenteral anticoagulant, begin edoxaban Wt >60 kg: 60 mg PO daily Wt ≤60 kg: 30 mg PO daily	CrCl >95: consider to avoid use CrCl 15–50: 30 mg PO daily CrCl <15: avoid use Not dialyzable Concomitant P-gp inhibitors (e.g., verapamil, quinidine, azithromycin, clarithromycin,	Avoid use with combined CYP3A4 and P-gp inducers (e.g., rifampin, phenytoin, carbamazepine, St. John's wort)

Continued

Table 24.6 Direct Oral Anticoagulants (DOACs)—cont'd

DRUG FORM	STANDARD DOSING	RENAL DOSING (USE ACTUAL WEIGHT FOR CrCl)	DRUG INTERACTION
		erythromycin, oral itraconazole, oral ketoconazole): 30 mg PO daily	Avoid use with combined CYP3A4 and P-gp inducers (e.g., rifampin, phenytoin, carbamazepine, St. John's wort)
Rivaroxaban (Xarelto) 2.5 mg, 10 mg, 15 mg, 20 mg	15 mg BID ×21 days, then 20 mg daily Take with food to increase bioavailability	CrCl <30: avoid use	Avoid use with combined strong CYP3A4 and P-gp inhibitors (e.g., ketoconazole, itraconazole, ritonavir)

Notes:

- For initial therapy, reserve apixaban and rivaroxaban only for hemodynamically stable patients without extensive clot burden; otherwise initiate parenteral anticoagulant then transition to apixaban or rivaroxaban
- Concurrent aspirin or thienopyridine increases bleeding
- Avoid prasugrel and ticagrelor
- Triple therapy (aspirin + thienopyridine + DOAC) increases bleeding and is not recommended

BID, Twice daily; *CrCl,* Creatinine clearance; *CYP,* Cytochrome P450 enzymes; *DOAC,* Direct oral anticoagulant; *P-gp,* P-glycoprotein; *PO,* Orally; *SCr,* Serum creatinine; *wt,* Weight

Data from Ageno W, Gallus AS, Wittkowsky A, et al. Oral anticoagulant therapy: antithrombotic therapy and prevention of thrombosis, 9th ed: American College of Chest Physicians evidence-based clinical practice guidelines. *Chest.* 2012;141(2 suppl):e44S–e88S; and from Kearon C, Akl EA, Ornelas J, et al. Antithrombotic therapy for VTE disease: chest guideline and expert panel report. *Chest.* 2016; 149(2):315–352.

- Initial dose: 5–10 mg daily for 2 days, then titrate to maintain international normalized ratio (INR) 2–3 for most indications (2.5–3.5 for mechanical heart valves)
- Consider lower initial dose if:
  - Elderly
  - Malnourished
  - Heart failure
  - Liver disease
  - Baseline INR elevated or high bleeding risk
  - Drug interaction that may potentiate warfarin
- Continue UFH/LWMH until INR therapeutic
- Drug interactions (Table 24.7)
- Fondaparinux
  - Factor Xa inhibitor
  - Useful for history of heparin-induced thrombocytopenia
  - Dosing
    - <50 kg: 5 mg subcutaneous (SubQ) daily
    - 50–100 kg: 7.5 mg SubQ daily
    - >100 kg: 10 mg SubQ daily
- Thrombolytic agents for acute PE (Table 24.8)
- Contraindications to thrombolytics (Table 24.9)
- Anticoagulation reversal agents and antidotes (Table 24.10)

Table 24.7 Significant Drug Interactions With Warfarin[a]

CLASS	DRUG	EFFECT ON WARFARIN
Antiarrhythmics	Amiodarone Dronedarone	↑ INR/risk of bleeding
Anti-infectives	Azole antifungals Cephalosporins (second and third generation) Fluoroquinolones Isoniazid Macrolides Metronidazole Penicillins (except for dicloxacillin/nafcillin) Sulfonamides Telithromycin Tetracyclines	↑ INR/risk of bleeding
	Griseofulvin Dicloxacillin/nafcillin Rifampin Rifabutin	↓ Anticoagulant effect
Anticoagulants	Apixaban Dabigatran Heparin/LMWH Rivaroxaban	↑ Anticoagulant effect

Antiepileptics	Carbamazepine	↓ Anticoagulant effect
	Phenytoin (chronic use)	
Antiplatelets	Aspirin	↑ Risk of bleeding
	Clopidogrel	
Herbals and supplements	Coenzyme Q10	↓ INR/bleed risk
	Ginseng	↓ Anticoagulant effect
	St. John's wort	
Nonsteroidal anti-inflammatory drugs (NSAIDs)	Ibuprofen	↑ INR/risk of bleeding
	Naproxen	
	COX-2 selective NSAIDs	
Pain medications	Tramadol	↑ INR/risk of bleeding
	Acetaminophen (>2 g/day)	
Selective serotonin reuptake inhibitors (SSRIs)	Fluoxetine	↑ INR/risk of bleeding
	Citalopram	
	Escitalopram	
	Sertraline	
	Paroxetine	

*The table is not all inclusive of potential drug interactions
INR, International normalized ratio; *LMWH*, Low-molecular-weight heparin
From Ageno W, Gallus AS, Witkowsky A, et al. Oral anticoagulant therapy: antithrombotic therapy and prevention of thrombosis, 9th ed: American College of Chest Physicians evidence-based clinical practice guidelines. *Chest.* 2012;141(2 Suppl):e44S–e88S.

Table 24.8 Thrombolytic Agents for Acute PE

| DRUG | STANDARD DOSING (IV) | | COMMENTS |
	INITIAL	MAINTENANCE	
Alteplase (Activase)	100 mg infused over 2 h	N/A	Fibrin selective Half-life: 5 min
Tenecteplase (TNKase)	<60 kg: 30 mg push 60–69 kg: 35 mg push 70–79 kg: 40 mg push 80–89 kg: 45 mg push ≥90 kg: 50 mg push	N/A	Fibrin selective (14-fold) Half-life: 90–130 min Only need bolus dose
Streptokinase Not available in U.S.	250,000 units over 30 min	100,000 units/h × 24h[a]	Nonselective Antigenic
Urokinase Not available in U.S.	4400 units/kg over 10 min	4400 units/kg/h × 12 h	Nonselective Concentration too dilute

Notes:

- Systemic thrombolytics are recommended for PE with hypotension (SBP < 90) who do not have a high bleeding risk.
- Complications:
  - Major hemorrhage: 9–12%
  - Intracranial hemorrhage: 1–2%
- Continuous-infusion heparin is used during thrombolytic therapy although it is frequently stopped and restarted after the completion of thrombolytic.

[a] 72h if concurrent deep vein thrombosis

IV, Intravenous; *N/A*, not applicable; *PE*, Pulmonary embolism; *SBP*, Systolic blood pressure

From Kearon C, Akl EA, Ornelas J, et al. Antithrombotic therapy for VTE disease: CHEST guideline and expert panel report. *Chest*. 2016; 149(2):315–352.

Table 24.9 Contraindications to Thrombolytic Agents for VTE

Absolute Contraindications

- History of intracranial hemorrhage
- Known structural intracranial disease
- Known malignant intracranial neoplasm
- Previous ischemic stroke within 3 months
- Active bleeding or bleeding diathesis
- Significant head trauma or facial trauma within 3 months
- Recent brain or spinal surgery

Relative Contraindications

- Severe uncontrolled hypertension on presentation (SBP >180 mm Hg or DBP >110 mm Hg)
- History of ischemic stroke more than 3 months prior
- Traumatic CPR or major surgery less than 3 weeks
- Recent internal bleeding within 2–4 weeks
- Noncompressible vascular punctures
- Recent invasive procedure
- Pregnancy
- Active peptic ulcer
- Pericarditis or pericardial fluid
- Current use of anticoagulant (e.g., warfarin) that has produced an elevated INR >1.7 or PT >15 s
- Age >75 years
- Diabetic retinopathy

CPR, Cardiopulmonary resuscitation; *DBP,* Diastolic blood pressure; *INR,* International normalized ratio; *PT,* Prothrombin time; *SBP,* Systolic blood pressure; *VTE,* Venous thromboembolism
Reproduced with permission from Kearon et al.[9]

Adapted from Kearon C, Akl EA, Ornelas J, et al. Antithrombotic therapy for VTE disease: CHEST guideline and expert panel report. *Chest.* 2016;149(2):315–352.

Table 24.10 Anticoagulation Reversal and Antidotes

AGENT FORM	STANDARD DOSING	PK/PD	COMMENT
Feiba (activated PCC) Factors II, IX, X, and activated factor VII	Off-label use: 25–100 units/kg IV (max: 200 units/kg/day) Rate not to exceed 2 units/kg/min	Onset: 15–30 min Duration: 8–12 h t ½: 4–7 h	To reverse DOAC Do not give within 12 h aminocaproic acid Factors II, IX, and X are nonactivated
Kcentra (Factors II, VII, IX, X, and antithrombotic proteins C and S and heparin)	Warfarin reversal: INR 2–4: 25 units/kg IV (max 2500 units) INR 4–6: 35 units/kg IV (max 3500 units) INR >6: 50 units/kg IV (max 5000 units)	Onset: rapid Duration: 6–8 h	Clotting factors are nonactivated Contains a small amount of heparin (allergy risk)
BebulinVH, Profilnine SD Three-factor (II, IX, X) PCC	Off-label use: INR <2: 20 units/kg IV INR 2–4: 30 units/kg IV INR >4: 50 units/kg IV ICH associated with warfarin: INR ≥1.4: 50 units/kg IV	Onset: 10–15 min Duration: 12–24 h	To reverse warfarin Clotting factors are nonactivated Contains a small amount of heparin (allergy risk)
Novoseven (recombinant human factor VIIa)	10–100 mcg/kg q2h until hemostasis achieved IV bolus over 2–5 min	Onset: 10 min Duration: 4–6 h	Lack of data for use in warfarin reversal; not recommended as monotherapy unless no alternative Not a blood product Short duration of action

Fresh frozen plasma (Octaplas)	10–15 mL/kg IV	Onset: 1–4 h Duration: 6 h	To replace human plasma proteins Thaw before use Avoid shaking Rate: <1 mL/kg/min with filter Give with NS flush
Protamine to reverse LMWH	IV protamine dosing (max 50 mg): If enoxaparin given in previous 8 h: protamine mg for mg of enoxaparin dose If enoxaparin given previous 8–12 h: protamine 0.5 mg for 1 mg of enoxaparin dose If last enoxaparin dose >3–5 t ½: protamine not recommended Other LMWH: If last LMWH dose within 3–5 t ½: protamine 0.5 mg for 100 anti-Xa units of LMWH	Onset: 5 min t ½: 7 min	Protamine has variable efficacy in reversing LMWH Max: 50 mg over 10 min to minimize risk of hypotension and bradycardia

Continued

Table 24.10 Anticoagulation Reversal and Antidotes—cont'd

AGENT FORM	STANDARD DOSING	PK/PD	COMMENT
Protamine to reverse UFH	IV protamine dosing for IV bolus heparin: If only a few min elapsed: 1 mg protamine per 100 units heparin If 30 min elapsed: 0.5 mg protamine per 100 units heparin If ≥2 h elapsed: 0.25–0.375 mg protamine per 100 units heparin For continuous-infusion heparin, use heparin dose infused over prior 2 h and give 1 mg protamine per 100 units heparin infused	Onset: 5 min t ½: 7 min	Heparin can be rapidly reversed with protamine Max: 50 mg over 10 min to minimize risk of hypotension and bradycardia IV use only
Vitamin K (phytonadione) Promotes liver synthesis of clotting factors	INR 4.5–10 (no bleed): none INR >10 (no bleed): 2.5–5 mg PO Minor bleed at any INR: 2.5–5 mg PO Major bleed: 5–10 mg IVPB in addition to four-factor PCC	Onset: 4–12 h Duration: PO: 6–10 h; 24–48 h for INR to normalize IVPB: 1–2 h; 12–14 h for INR to normalize t ½: 26–193 h	To reverse warfarin IM: avoid, risk of hematoma IV push: avoid, risk of anaphylaxis/hypotension SubQ: variable absorption PO: preferred if no bleeding IVPB: 1–10 mg in 50 mL over 30 min May repeat PO dose after 24 h if INR not corrected May repeat IV dose after 12 h if INR not corrected

Idarucizumab (Praxbind) (humanized monoclonal antibody fragment)	Reversal of dabigatran: IV 2.5 g ×2 no more than 15 min apart	Onset: min Duration: 24 h t ½: Initial: 7 min Terminal: 10 h	To reverse dabigatran Do not combine with PCC Do not mix or run with any other IV solution
Andexanet alfa (Andexxa)	Apixaban or rivaroxaban >7 h: IV 400 mg bolus then 4 mg/min ×120 min Enoxaparin, edoxaban, rivaroxaban within 7 h or unknown time: IV 800 mg bolus then 8 mg/min ×120 min	Onset: rapid Duration: 2 h t ½: 1 h	To reverse DOAC
Tranexamic acid (Cyklop-aron)	PO: 1–1.5 g q8–12h IV: 10–20 mg/kg ×1 bolus then 10 mg/kg Q6–8h	Time to peak: IV: 5 min PO: 3 h Duration: IV: 17 h PO: 24 h t ½: 2–11 h	Competitive inhibitor of plasmin and plasminogen
Aminocaproic acid (Amicar)	IV: 2 g q6h	Onset: 1–72 h t ½: 1–2 h	10-Fold weaker than tranexamic acid Hypotension and bradycardia with rapid infusion Rhabdomyolysis

Continued

Table 24.10 Anticoagulation Reversal and Antidotes—cont'd

AGENT FORM	STANDARD DOSING	PK/PD	COMMENT
Oral activated charcoal	PO: 25–100 g ×1 or 50–100 g ×1 followed by 25–50 g q4h	n/a	Use if last dabigatran dose within 2 h Use if last rivaroxaban dose within 8 h Use if last apixaban or edoxaban dose within 6 h

DOAC, Direct oral anticoagulant; *ICH,* Intracranial hemorrhage; *IM,* Intramuscularly; *INR,* International normalized ratio; *IV,* Intravenously; *IVPB,* IV piggy back; *LMWH,* Low-molecular-weight heparin; max: Maximum; *PCC,* Prothrombin complex concentrate; *PD/PK,* Pharmacodynamics/pharmacokinetics; *PO,* Orally; *SubQ,* Subcutaneous; *t ½,* Half-life elimination; *UFH,* Unfractionated heparin

From Ageno W, Gallus AS, Witkowsky A, et al. Oral anticoagulant therapy: antithrombotic therapy and prevention of thrombosis, 9th ed: American College of Chest Physicians evidence-based clinical practice guidelines. *Chest.* 2012;141(2 SUPPL):e44S–e88S.

References

1. Goldhaber SZ. Risk factors for venous thromboembolism. *J Am Coll Cardiol.* 2010;56(1):1–7.
2. Lijfering WM, Rosendaal FR, Cannegieter SC. Risk factors for venous thrombosis—current understanding from an epidemiological point of view. *Br J Haematol.* 2010;149(6):824–833.
3. Spencer FA, Emery C, Lessard D, et al. The Worcester Venous Thrombo-embolism Study: a population-based study of the clinical epidemiology of venous thromboembolism. *J Gen Intern Med.* 2006;21:722–727.
4. Falck-Ytter Y, Francis CW, Johanson NA, et al. Prevention of VTE in ortho-pedic surgery patients. *Chest.* 2012;141(2 suppl):e278S–e325S.
5. Gould MK, Garcia DA, Wren SM, et al. Prevention of VTE in nonorthopedic surgical patients. *Chest.* 2012;141(2 suppl):e227S–e277S.
6. Guyatt GH, Akl EA, Crowther M, Gutterman DD, Schünemann HJ. Execu-tive summary antithrombotic therapy and prevention of thrombosis, 9th ed: American College of Chest Physicians evidence-based clinical practice guidelines. *Chest.* 2012;141(2 suppl):7S–47S.
7. Holbrook A, Schulman S, Witt DM, et al. Evidence-based management of anticoagulant therapy: antithrombotic therapy and prevention of throm-bosis, 9th ed: American College of Chest Physicians evidence-based clinical practice guidelines. *Chest.* 2012;141(2 Suppl):e152S–e184S.
8. Ageno W, Gallus AS, Wittkowsky A, Crowther M, Hylek EM, Palareti G. Oral anticoagulant therapy: antithrombotic therapy and prevention of thrombosis, 9th ed: American College of Chest Physicians evidence-based clinical practice guidelines. *Chest.* 2012;141(2 suppl):e44S–e88S.
9. Kearon C, Akl EA, Ornelas J, et al. Antithrombotic therapy for VTE disease: CHEST guideline and expert panel report. *Chest.* 2016;149(2):315–352.

Appendix

Drugs Associated With Fever

Allopurinol	Azathioprine	β lactams	Bleomycin
Chemotherapy agents	Diltiazem	Diuretics	Fluoroquinolones
H_2 antihistamine	Haloperidol	Hydralazine	Interferon-α
Interleukin-2	Minocycline	Narcotics	Procainamide
Quinidine	Rifampin	SSRIs	Succinylcholine
Sulfonamides	Tacrolimus	Thyroxine	TMP-SMX

SSRIs, Serotonin reuptake inhibitors; *TMP/SMX,* Trimethoprim-sulfamethoxazole
Data from Ferri FF. *Ferri's Clinical Advisor.* Philadelphia: Elsevier; 2020:1538–1545; Rosmarin C, Jawad A. *Hutchison's Clinical Methods.* Philadelphia: Elsevier; 2018:141–155; and Cunha BA. *Infect Dis Clin N Am.* 2007;21(4):867–915.

Drugs Associated With Neutropenia

ACE inhibitors	Adalimumab	Allopurinol	Amphotericin
β-Blockers	Carbamazepine	Cephalosporins	Chemotherapy agents
Chloramphenicol	Chloroquine	Chlorpromazine	Clozapine
Corticosteroids	Cyclosporine	Dapsone	Deferasirox
Deferiprone	Diclofenac	Digoxin	Dipyridamole
Diuretics	Etanercept	Ethosuximide	Flecainide
Flucytosine	Ganciclovir	Gold salts	H_2 antihistamine
Ibuprofen	Indomethacin	Leflunomide	Linezolid
Macrolides	Mefloquine	Methimazole	Nifedipine
Olanzapine	Penicillins	Phenothiazines	Phenytoin
Procainamide	Propylthiouracil	Quinine	Rituximab
Salicylates	Sirolimus	Sulfasalazine	Sulfonamides
Sulfonylureas	Tacrolimus	Tetracyclines	Tricyclic agents
Valacyclovir	Valproic acid	Vancomycin	

ACE, Angiotensin-converting enzyme
Data from Callandar NS. *Conn's Current Therapy.* Philadelphia: Elsevier; 2019:429–434; Rice L, Jung M. *Hematology: Basic Principles and Practice.* Philadelphia: Elsevier; 2018:675–681, chap 48; and Maciejewski JP, Thota S. *Hematology: Basic Principles and Practice.* Philadelphia: Elsevier; 2018: 425–444.e5, chap 32.

Drugs Associated With Thrombocytopenia

Acetaminophen	Aminoglutethimide	Amiodarone	Amphotericin B
Antiplatelet agents	Barbiturates	Captopril	Carbamazepine
Cephalosporins	Chloramphenicol	Chloroquine	Chlorothiazide
Chlorpropamide	Codeine	Cyclophospha-mide	Danazol
Desipramine	Diazepam	Diazoxide	Digoxin
Erythromycin	Estrogen	Ethambutol	Fluconazole
Fluorouracil	Gemcitabine	Gentamicin	Gold salts
H$_2$ blockers	Haloperidol	Heparins[a]	Imipenem
Interferon alfa	Isoniazid	Lansoprazole	Levodopa
Lidocaine	Linezolid	Lithium	Meperidine
Meprobamate	Mesalamine	Minoxidil	Methimazole
Methotrexate	Methyldopa	Nitroglycerin	NSAIDs
Omeprazole	Oxaliplatin	Pantoprazole	Penicillamine
Penicillins	Pentoxifylline	Phenothiazines	Phenytoin
Prednisone	Procarbazine	Propylthiouracil	Protease inhibitors
Quinidine	Quinine	Rabeprazole	Rifampin
Statins	Streptomycin	Sulfonamides	Tamoxifen
Tetracyclines	TMP/SMX	Tolbutamide	Valproic acid
Vancomycin			

NSAID, Nonsteroidal anti-inflammatory drug; *TMP/SMX,* Trimethoprim-sulfamethoxazole
[a]Unfractionated and low-molecular-weight

Data from James WD, Elston DM, Treat JR, Rosenbach MA, Neuhaus IM. *Andrews' Diseases of the Skin.* Philadelphia: Elsevier; 2020:35, 813–861.e5; Scott JP, Flood VH. *Nelson Textbook of Pediatrics.* Philadelphia: Elsevier; 2020: 2609–2618.e3, chap 511;and Taira T. *Emergency Medicine.* Philadelphia: Elsevier; 2013:205, 1714–1720.e1.

Therapeutic Drug Levels

DRUG	THERAPEUTIC RANGE	TIMING OF LEVEL
Amikacin peak	20–35 mcg/mL	30 min after infusion
Amikacin trough	<10 mcg/mL	Just prior to next dose
Amitriptyline + nortriptyline	95–250 ng/mL	Just prior to next dose
Carbamazepine trough	4–12 mcg/mL	Just prior to next dose
Cyclosporine trough	100–400 ng/mL	Just prior to next dose
Desipramine	100–300 ng/mL	Just prior to next dose
Digoxin trough	0.8–2 ng/mL Heart failure: 0.5–0.9 ng/mL	Just prior to next dose
Disopyramide	2–6 mcg/mL	Just prior to next dose
Ethosuximide trough	40–100 mcg/mL	Just prior to next dose
Gentamicin peak	5–10 mcg/mL	30 min after infusion
Gentamicin trough	<2 mcg/mL	Just prior to next dose
Imipramine trough	150–200 ng/mL	Just prior to next dose
Lidocaine	1.2–5 mcg/mL	12–24 h after start of infusion
Lithium trough	0.6–1.2 meq/L	Just prior to next dose
Nortriptyline trough	50–150 ng/mL	Just prior to next dose
Phenobarbital trough	15–40 mcg/mL	Just prior to next dose
Phenytoin trough	Total: 10–20 mcg/mL Free: 1–2.5 mcg/mL	Just prior to next dose
Primidone trough	5–12 mcg/mL	Just prior to next dose
Procainamide	4–10 mcg/mL	Just prior to next dose
Quinidine	1.5–4.5 mcg/mL	Just prior to next dose
Theophylline	10–20 mcg/mL	8–12 h after once-daily dose

Continued

Therapeutic Drug Levels—cont'd

DRUG	THERAPEUTIC RANGE	TIMING OF LEVEL
Tobramycin peak	5–10 mcg/mL	30 min after infusion
Tobramycin trough	<2 mcg/mL	Just prior to next dose
Valproate trough	Epilepsy: 50–100 mcg/mL Mania: 45–125 mcg/mL	Just prior to next dose
Vancomycin trough	10–20 mcg/mL	Just prior to next dose

From Kratz A, Pesce MA. *Goldman-Cecil Medicine*. Philadelphia: Elsevier; 2020.

Opioid Conversion

OPIOID	APPROXIMATE EQUIANALGESIC DOSE (mg)		USUAL STARTING DOSE	
	PARENTERAL	ORAL	PARENTERAL	ORAL
Morphine	10	30	3 mg q4h	10 mg q4h
Codeine	—	200	—	30 mg q4h
Fentanyl	0.1	—	0.1 mg q1h	—
Hydrocodone	—	30	—	10 mg q4–6h
Hydromorphone	1.5	7.5	0.4 mg q2h	2 mg q4h
Oxycodone	—	20	—	10 mg q4–6h
Oxymorphone	1 mg	10	1 mg q4–6h	5 mg q4–6h
Tramadol	—	300 mg	—	50 mg q4–6h

Notes:
- Opioid dosage conversions are only estimates, thus do not consider patient variability in clinical response
- Consider reducing converted opioid dose by 25–50% initially then titrate as appropriate

From Anthony A. *Ferri's Clinical Advisor*. Philadelphia: Elsevier; 2019.

Morphine to Fentanyl Patch Conversion

ORAL MORPHINE EQUIVALENT (mg/24 h)	FENTANYL TRANSDERMAL PATCH (mcg/h)
60–134	25
135–224	50
225–314	75
315–404	100

Notes:
- Onset of pain relief is delayed approximately 12 h, with its peak effect in 20–72 h; thus, rescue opioids should be provided during the first 24 h of fentanyl patch
- Transdermal patch is not recommended in the following:
  - Sepsis
  - Acute pain
  - Cachexia
  - Significant dermatologic insults

From DURAGESIC(R) transdermal system, fentanyl transdermal system [product information]. Titusville, NJ: Janssen Pharmaceuticals Inc (per manufacturer); 2018.

References

1. Ferri FF. *Ferri's Clinical Advisor*. Philadelphia: Elsevier; 2020:1538–1545.
2. Rosmarin C, Jawad A. *Hutchison's Clinical Methods*. Philadelphia: Elsevier; 2018:141–155.
3. Cunha BA. Fever of unknown origin: clinical overview of classic and current concepts. *Infect Dis Clin N Am*. 2007;21(4):867–915.
4. Callandar NS. *Conn's Current Therapy*. Philadelphia: Elsevier; 2019:429–434.
5. Rice L, Jung M. *Hematology: Basic Principles and Practice*. Philadelphia: Elsevier; 2018:675–681, chap 48.
6. Maciejewski JP, Thota S. *Hematology: Basic Principles and Practice*. Philadelphia: Elsevier; 2018:425–444.e5, chap 32.
7. James WD, Elston DM, Treat JR, Rosenbach MA, Neuhaus IM. *Andrews' Diseases of the Skin*. Philadelphia: Elsevier; 2020:35, 813–861.e5.
8. Scott JP, Flood VH. *Nelson Textbook of Pediatrics*. Philadelphia: Elsevier; 2020:2609–2618.e3, chap 511.
9. Taira T. *Emergency Medicine*. Philadelphia: Elsevier; 2013:205, 1714–1720.e1.
10. Kratz A, Pesce MA. *Goldman-Cecil Medicine*. Philadelphia: Elsevier; 2020:e1–e10, appendix.
11. Anthony A. *Ferri's Clinical Advisor*. Philadelphia: Elsevier; 2020:1016–1018.e2.
12. DURAGESIC(R) transdermal system, fentanyl transdermal system [product information]. Titusville, NJ: Janssen Pharmaceuticals Inc. (per manufacturer); 2018.

Index

Page numbers followed by *f* indicate figures, *t* indicate tables, *b* indicate boxes.